WHAT'S NEW IN ANESTHESIOLOGY

DEVELOPMENTS IN CRITICAL CARE MEDICINE AND ANESTHESIOLOGY

Prakash, O. (ed.): Applied Physiology in Clinical Respiratory Care. 1982. ISBN 90-247-2662-X.

McGeown, Mary G.: Clinical Management of Electrolyte Disorders. 1983. ISBN 0-89838-559-8.

Scheck, P.A., Sjöstrand, U.H., and Smith, R.B. (eds.): Perspectives in High Frequency Ventilation. 1983. ISBN 0-89838-571-7.

Stanley, T.H., and Petty, W.C. (eds.): New Anesthetic Agents, Devices and Monitoring Techniques. 1983. ISBN 0-89838-566-0.

Prakash, O. (ed.): Computing in Anesthesia and Intensive Care. 1983. ISBN 0-89838-602-0.

Stanley, T.H., and Petty, W.C. (eds.): Anesthesia and the Cardiovascular System. 1984. ISBN 0-89838-626-8.

Van Kleef, J.W., Burm, A.G.L., and Spierdijk, J. (eds.): Current Concepts in Regional Anaesthesia. 1984. ISBN 0-89838-644-6.

Prakash, O. (ed.): Critical Care of the Child. 1984. ISBN 0-89838-661-6.

Stanley, T.H., and Petty, W.C. (eds.): Anesthesiology: Today and Tomorrow. 1985. ISBN 0-89838-705-1.

Rahn, H., and Prakash, O. (eds.): Acid-base Regulation and Body Temperature. 1985. ISBN 0-89838-708-6.

Stanley, T.H., and Petty, W.C. (eds.): Anesthesiology 1986. 1986. ISBN 0-89838-779-5.

de Lange, S., Hennis, P.J., and Kettler, D. (eds.): Cardiac Anaesthesia: Problems and Innovations. 1986. ISBN 0-89838-794-9.

Stanley, T.H., and Petty, W.C. (eds.): Anesthesia, the Heart and the Vascular System. 1987. ISBN 0-89838-851-1.

Stanley, T.H. (ed.): What's New in Anesthesiology. 1988. ISBN 0-89838-367-6.

WHAT'S NEW IN ANESTHESIOLOGY

edited by

T.H. STANLEY

Department of Anesthesiology,
The University of Utah Medical School,
Salt Lake City, USA

1988 **MARTINUS NIJHOFF PUBLISHERS**
a member of the KLUWER ACADEMIC PUBLISHERS GROUP
DORDRECHT / BOSTON / LANCASTER

Distributors

for the United States and Canada: Kluwer Academic Publishers, 101 Philip Drive, Assinippi Park, Norwell, MA 02061, USA
for the UK and Ireland: Kluwer Academic Publishers, MTP Press Limited, Falcon House, Queen Square, Lancaster LA1 1RN, UK
for all other countries: Kluwer Academic Publishers Group, Distribution Center, P.O. Box 322, 3300 AH Dordrecht, The Netherlands

Library of Congress Cataloging in Publication Data

What's new in anesthesiology.

(Developments in critical care medicine and anaesthesiology)
"Presentations of the 33rd Annual Postgraduate Course in Anesthesiology which took place ... in Salt Lake City, Utah, February 19-23, 1988"--Pref.
Includes bibliographies.
1. Anesthesiology--Congresses. 2. Medical innovations--Congresses. I. Stanley, Theodore H. (Theodore, Henry), 1940- . II. Utah Postgraduate Course in Anesthesiology (33rd : 1988 : Salt Lake City, Utah) III. Series. [DNLM: 1. Anesthesiology--congresses. W3 UT294 33rd 1988 / WO 200 W555 1988]
RD78.4.W47 1988 617'.96 87-34751

ISBN-13: 978-94-010-7713-2 e-ISNB-13: 978-94-009-2689-9
DOI: 10.1007/978-94-009-2689-9

Copyright

PREFACE

Theodore H. Stanley, M.D.

What's New in Anesthesiology in 1988 contains the Refresher Course manuscripts of the presentations of the 33rd Annual Postgraduate Course in Anesthesiology which took place at the Marriott Hotel Convention Center in Salt Lake City, Utah, February 19-23, 1988. The chapters reflect new data, ideas and concepts within the general framework of most recent developments in "evaluation and monitoring cardiac function before, during and after surgery," "new anesthetics and their actions on the heart and peripheral vasculature, and other organ systems," "metabolism and elimination of anesthetics and anesthetic adjuvants," and "recent developments in the anesthetic management of patients with congenital heart disease, renal and pulmonary dysfunction, and diabetes insipidus." In addition, there are chapters on new developments in "obstetrics," "regional anesthesia," and "anesthetic management of the newborn." The purposes of the textbook are to 1) act as a reference for the anesthesiologists attending the meeting, and 2) serve as a vehicle to bring many of the latest concepts in anesthesiology to others within a short time of the formal presentation. Each chapter is a brief but sharply focused glimpse of the interests in anesthesia expressed at the conference. This book and its chapters should not be considered complete treatises on the subjects addressed but rather attempts to summarize the most salient points. This textbook is the sixth in a continuing series documenting the proceedings of the Postgraduate Course in Salt Lake City. We hope that this and the past and future volumes reflect the rapid and continuing evolution of anesthesiology in the late twentieth century.

TABLE OF CONTENTS

LIST OF CONTRIBUTORS

Bailey, P.L.
Department of Anesthesiology, The University of Utah School of Medicine, Salt Lake City, UT 84132, U.S.A.

Barash, P.
Department of Anesthesiology, Yale University School of Medicine, New Haven, CT 06510, U.S.A.

Clark, N.J.
Department of Anesthesiology, University of Utah School of Medicine, Salt Lake City, UT 84132, U.S.A.

Foëx, P.
Nuffield Department of Anesthetics, The Radcliffe Infirmary, Oxford OX2 6HE, United Kingdom

Joyce, T.H.
Department of Anesthesiology, Jefferson Davis Hospital, Baylor College of Medicine, Houston, TX 77019, U.S.A.

Merin, R.
Department of Anesthesiology, University of Texas, Medical School at Houston, Houston, TX 77004, U.S.A.

Savarese, J.J.
Department of Anesthesia, Massachusetts General Hospital, Boston, MA 02114, U.S.A.

Schwartz, A.J.
Associate Dean for Academic Affairs, Hahnemann University, Philadelphia, PA 19102, U.S.A.

Tonnesen, A.S.
Department of Anesthesiology, University of Texas Health Science Center at Houston, Houston, TX 77004, U.S.A.

Winnie, A.P.
Department of Anesthesiology, University of Illinois College of Medicine at Chicago, 1740 West Traylor Street, Chicago, IL 60612, U.S.A.

UNDERSTANDING LEFT VENTRICULAR FUNCTION

P.FOËX and B.LEONE

The characteristics of cardiac muscle contraction and relaxation have been extensively investigated using isolated heart muscle preparations. In such preparations, the effects of changes in preload (Starling's law of the heart) and in contractility have been clearly defined, and many indices of contractility described. These indices, extensively validated in isolated heart muscle preparations, have been used to assess the inotropic state of the intact heart. However, the intact heart is not a band of muscle lifting a weight, it is a muscle pump ejecting a viscous fluid (the blood) into viscoelastic systems (the systemic and pulmonary circulations). In order to characterize the behaviour of the cardiac pump, the dynamic relationships between pressure and dimensions may be more appropriate than the analysis of pressure alone.

Pressure-dimensions relationships:

The idea of representing ventricular contraction and relaxation in terms of the instantaneous relationship between pressure and volume is not new. Frank described such a relationship for the frog heart in 1895 (1). Pressure-dimension loops can be constructed for the ejecting ventricle if, besides intraventricular pressure, volume, diameter, or myocardial chord length are measured throughout the cardiac cycle (2,3,4). The loop consists of four segments, representing isovolumic contraction, ejection, isovolumic relaxation, and ventricular filling; these are delineated by four events: mitral valve closure, aortic valve opening, aortic valve closure, and mitral valve opening (Fig 1).

The effect of volume loading is to displace the end-diastolic point of the loop along the end-diastolic pressure dimension line, which represents the static compliance of the ventricle (Fig 2). The line becomes steeper as loading increases.

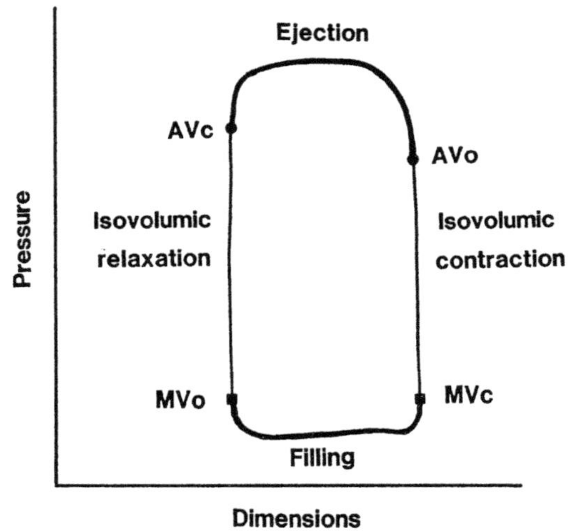

Figure 1. Diagrammatic representation of a pressure-dimension loop. The phases of the cardiac cycle are represented together with the times of mitral valve closure (MVc), aortic valve opening (AVo), aortic valve closure (AVc) and mitral valve opening (MVo).

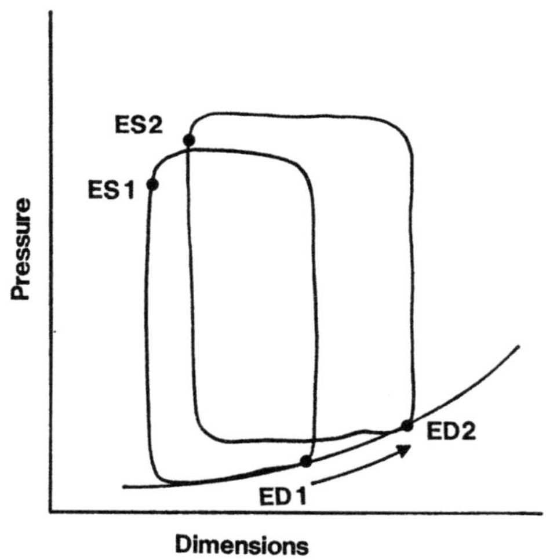

Figure 2. An increase in preload displaces the end-diastolic pressure-dimension point (ED1 to ED2) along the end-diastolic pressure-dimension line. Note that the displacement of end-systolic pressure-dimension point (ES1 to ES2) is much smaller, hence the increase in stroke volume (represented by the width of the loop).

As a volume load is administered, the end-systolic dimensions increase to a lesser extent than the end-diastolic dimensions, and the stroke volume increases.

Increases in the resistance to ejection displace the end-systolic points of the loop along a straight line, the end-systolic pressure-dimension line (5). As resistance increases, so do the end-systolic dimensions. Conversely, reductions in resistance allow the ventricle to contract to smaller end-systolic dimensions (Fig 3).

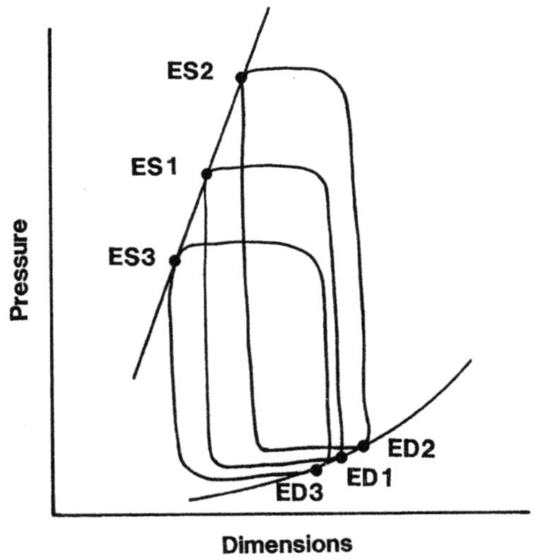

Figure 3. Changes in resistance to ejection cause a displacement of the end-systolic pressure-dimension point (ES1, ES2, ES3) along a straight line. Note that the end-diastolic pressure-dimension point is displaced to a much smaller extent, hence the changes in stroke volume caused by the changes in resistance.

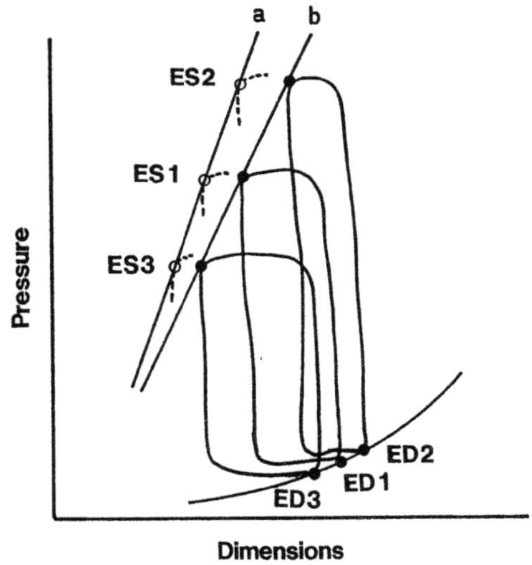

Figure 4. Negative inotropy causes flattening of the end-systolic pressure-dimension line (a to b). The width of the loop is reduced and the effects of changes in resistance exaggerated.

Changes in the inotropic state of the myocardium modify the slope of the end-systolic pressure-dimension line. Positive inotropic interventions increase, whilst negative inotropic interventions (Fig 4) decrease this slope.

The area of the pressure-volume loop represents the external work of the ventricle (6) for that beat (the stroke work), while the triangular area delineated by the end-systolic pressure-volume line, the end-diastolic pressure-volume line, and the loop represents the potential energy of the ventricle (Fig 5). The total free mechanical energy the ventricle liberates

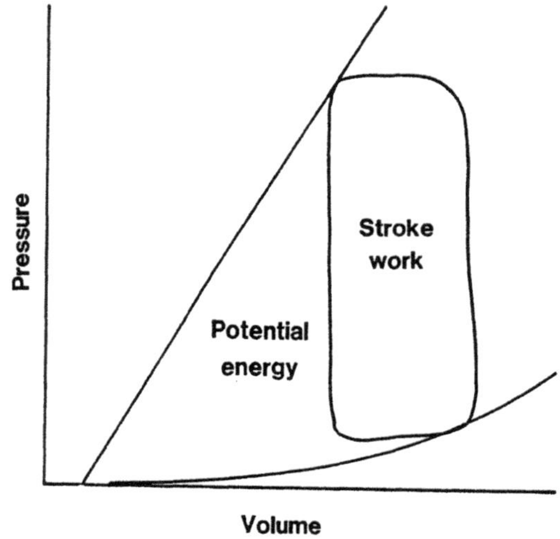

Figure 5. The area of the presure-volume loop represents the stroke work. The area to the left of the loop, delineated by the end-systolic and end-diastolic pressure-volume lines represents the potential energy of the heart.

during each contraction, for given preloads and afterloads, may be represented by the sum of the external work and potential energy. Indeed, a very high correlation has been observed between myocardial oxygen consumption and the sum of these areas of the pressure-volume loop (7).

With global left ventricular failure, the slope of the end-systolic pressure-dimension line becomes flatter, and the intercept of this line with the dimension axis (often termed V_d, the dead volume) becomes larger as the end-diastolic pressure-dimension line becomes steeper (8). These alterations modify the effects of changes in preload and afterload on left ventricular ejection. The failing heart ejects from larger end-diastolic dimensions (and, hence, from larger end-diastolic pressures) than the normal heart, and

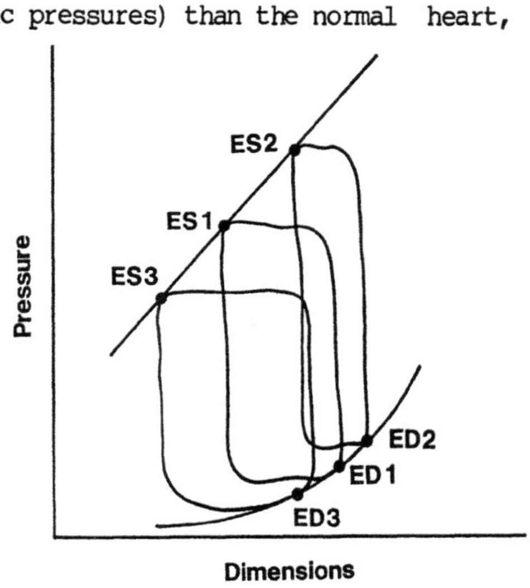

Figure 6. When the left ventricle is failing, the end-systolic pressure-dimension line is flatter, and the end-diastolic pressure-dimension line steeper than normal. Changes in resistance cause exaggerated changes in end-systolic dimensions and in end-diastolic pressure.

because of the reduced inotropic state, contracts less to larger end-systolic dimensions. Increases in vascular resistance cause exaggerated reductions in stroke volume, while vasodilatation enhances ejection (Fig 6).

Pressure-length relationship:

Because of the segmental nature of coronary artery disease, assessment of global ventricular performance may not be as informative as assessment of regional wall motion. Indeed, studies using radionuclides, echocardiography, and cardiokymography, have shown that coronary artery disease may cause moderate or severe impairment of regional wall function at rest or during exercise (9). Wall motion may be decreased (hypokinesia), abolished (akinesia), or become paradoxical (dyskinesia). Quite frequently wall motion is described in terms of extent of shortening (or extent of wall thickening if wall thickness is measured), attention being paid to abnormal patterns of wall motion (systolic lengthening, post-systolic shortening;10,11). However, examination of the pressure-length loop facilitates the detection of segmental abnormalities caused by asynchrony of contraction and relaxation.

Myocardial ischaemia causes marked alterations of the pressure-length loop (12,13). Moderate ischaemia causes the loop to lean to the right (Fig 7). This results from the lengthening of the ischaemic segment during isovolumic contraction, and from shortening during isovolumic relaxation (post-systolic shortening). Systolic lengthening represents the displacement forced upon the ischaemic segment by the normal adjoining segments. Such a

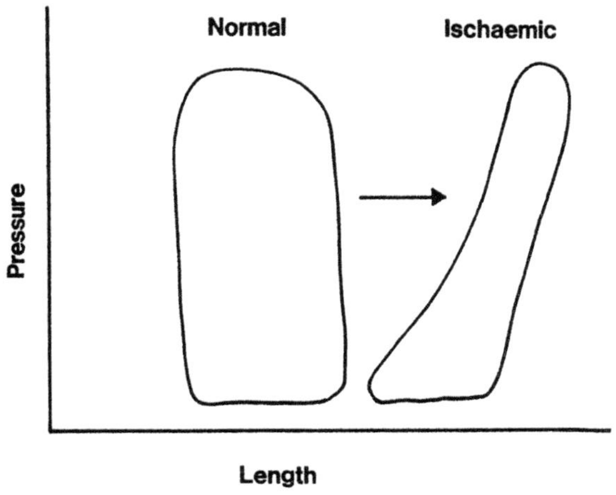

Figure 7. Myocardial ischaemia alters the shape of the pressure-length loop. The ischaemic segment dilates (rightward shift), exhibits paradoxical systolic lengthening (the loops leans to the right), shortens less during systole (the top of the loop is narrow), and continues to shorten after aortic valve closure (the foot ot the loop is wider than its top).

displacement may occur because of delayed electrical activation or because of a change in preload tension in the ischaemic region. Post-systolic shortening, previously attributed to the effect of elastic recoil, is almost certainly an active phenomenon. However, because it occurs after aortic valve closure, it does not contribute to ejection.

Recently, abnormal pressure-length relationships, very similar to those seen in ischaemic myocardium, have been observed in the apex of the left ventricle, in the absence of ischaemia, when calcium antagonists were adminstered together with halothane or isoflurane (14,15). This suggests that abnormal pressure-length loops may represent a state of asynchronous contraction that can be caused by ischaemia or by other interventions that uncouple excitation and contraction.

By analogy with the area of the pressure-volume loop, the area of the pressure-length loop may be used as an index of regional work. Interpretation of the area of the pressure-length loop is difficult when asynchrony of contraction is present. When the loop leans to the right, its area encompasses three distinct regions (Fig 8). The region corresponding to systolic lengthening represents work done <u>on</u> the segment by normal neighbouring segments, and not work done <u>by</u> the segment itself. The region delineated by post-systolic shortening represents work done by the segment but ineffective in terms of the overall pump function of the left ventricle because it occurs after aortic valve closure. Only the central region of the loop represents the effective contribution of the segment to the work of the left ventricle. The ratio of this area to the total area gives an estimate

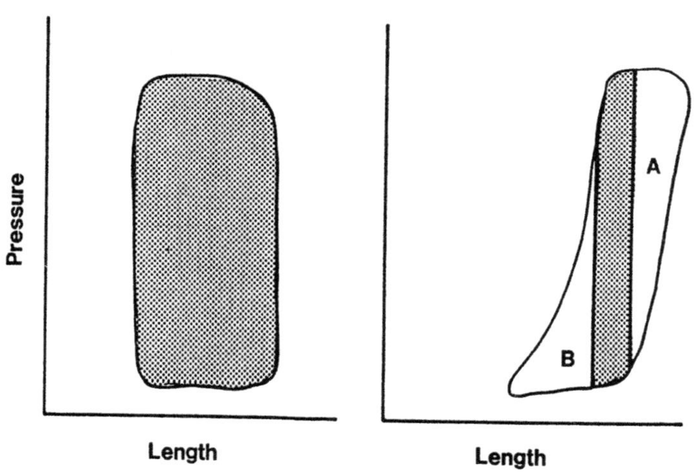

<u>Figure 8</u>. When a segment contracts normally (right hand panel) the loop is upright and its area (shaded) is an index of the contribution of the segment to the total stroke work. When ischaemia is present (left hand panel) the effective contribution (shaded area) is much smaller than the total loop area. The non-shaded areas (A,B) correspond to work done on the segment (A), or work that does not contribute to ejection (B).

of the effectiveness of segment. Ischaemia and asynchony of contraction caused by the association of calcium antagonists and inhalational anaesthetics reduce the effectiveness of contraction; when large areas of the left ventricle are involved, this will be reflected in poor global function.

The relationships between left ventricular presure and left ventricular dimensions or length can yield important information regarding the inotropic state of the left ventricle and encompass the concepts of potential energy as well as observed energy expendend in contraction. Presure-length relationships are also sensitive to regional ischaemic changes and drug-induced regional myocardial dysfunction. While such relationships may not be obtained clinically as easily as experimentally, they provide a framework for a better understanding of left ventricular function.

References:

1 Frank, O. (1895). Zur Dynamik des Herzmuskels. Z.Biol., **32**, 370-447.

2 Suga, H. (1969). Time course of left ventricular pressure-volume relationship under various end-distolic volumes. Jap.Heart J., **10**, 509-515.

3 Olsen, C.O., Tyson, G.S., Maier, G.W., Spratt, J.A., Davis, J.W., and Rankin, J.S. (1983). Dynamic ventricular interaction in the conscious dog. Circ.Res., **52**, 85-104

4 Theroux, P., Franklin, D., Ross, J. and Kemper, W.S. (1974). Regional myocardial function during acute coronary artery occlusion and its modification by pharmacologoic agents in the dog. Circ.Res., **35**, 896-908.

5 Mahler, F., Covell, J.W. and Ross, J. (1975). Systolic pressure-diameter relations in normal conscious dog. Cardiovasc.Res., **9**, 447-455.

6 Forrester, J.S., Tyberg, J.V., Wyatt, H.L., Goldner, S. Parmley, W.W. and Swan, H.J.C. (1974). Pressure-length loop: a new method for simultaneous measurement of segmental and total cardiac function. J.Appl.Physiol., **37**, 771-775.

7 Suga, H.,Hayashi, T., and Shirahata,M. (1981). Ventricular pressure volume area as predictor of cardiac oxygen consumption. Am.J.Physiol., **237**, H39-H44.

8 Grossman, W., Braunwald, E., Mann, T., McLaurin, L.P., and Green, L.H. (1977). Contractile state of the left ventricle in amn as evaluated from end-systolic pressure-volume relations. Circulation, **56**, 845-852.

9 Thys, D.M. (1987). The intraoperative assessment of regional myocardial performance: is the cart before the horse ? Cardiothor.Anesth., **1**, 273-275.

10 Bugge-Asperheim,B., Leraand,S. and Kiil,F.(1969). Local dimensional changes of the myocardium measured by ultrasonic technique. Scand.J.Clin.Lab.Invest.,**24**, 361-371.

11 Franklin, D., Kemper, W.S., Patrick, T. and McKown, D. (1973). Technique for continuous measurement of regional myocardial segment dimensions in chronic animal preparations. Fed.Proc., **32**, 343.

12 Theroux, P., Ross, J., Franklin, D., Kemper, W.S. and Sasayama, S. (1976). Regional myocardial function in the conscious dog during acute coronary occlusion and response to morphine, propranolol, nitroglycerin and lidocaine. Circulation, **53**, 302-314.

13 Doyle, R.L., Foëx, P., Ryder, W.A., and Jones, L.A. (1987) Differences in ischaemic dysfunction following gradual vs abrupt coronary occlusion: Effects on isovolumic relaxation. Cardiovas.Res., **21**, 507-514.

14 Ramsay, J.G., Cutfield, G.R., Francis, C.M., Devlin, W.H. and Foëx, P. (1986). Halothane-verapamil causes regional myocardial dysfunction in the dog. Br.J.Anaesth., **58**, 321-326.

15 Videcoq, M., Arvieux, C.C., Ramsay, J.G., Foëx, P., Stone, J.G., Ryder, W.A., and Jones, L.A. (1987) The association isoflurane-verapamil causes regional myocardial dysfunction. Anesthesiology, (In the Press).

MONITORING MYOCARDIAL OXYGEN BALANCE: PHYSIOLOGIC BASIS AND CLINICAL APPLICATION

P. BARASH

The development of therapeutic strategies to ensure a favorable balance between myocardial oxygen delivery (SUPPLY) and myocardial oxygen consumption (DEMAND) is mandatory for patients with coronary artery disease. Myocardial ischemia can lead to clinically significant circulatory impairment. Slogoff and Keats emphasized the importance of detection of perioperative ischemia in a study that related the incidence of ischemia to postoperative myocardial infarction.[1] Calculation of myocardial oxygen supply and consumption (MVO_2) requires the direct of measurement coronary blood flow.

Supply	Demand
Coronary O_2 transport = CBF x CaO_2	MVO_2 = CBF (CaO_2 - $CcsO_2$)

MVO_2 = Myocardial Oxygen Consumption
CBF = Coronary Blood Flow
CaO_2 = Arterial Oxygen Content
$CcsO_2$ = coronary sinus O_2 content

Routine measurement of coronary blood flow, such as thermodilution coronary sinus blood flow and sampling, is not feasible for general clinical application. Therefore, at present, the clinician must rely on various methods of indirectly assessing myocardial supply/demand relationships to aid in patient management. To better appreciate the limitations of these methods, brief consideration will be given to the physiology of coronary circulation.

I. THE CORONARY CIRCULATION

During systole a high wall tension is developed in the left ventricle. Extravascular compression of the subendocardial zone results in diversion of left ventricular coronary blood flow to the epicardial zone. This, in part, accounts for the vulnerability of sub-endocardium to ischemia. During diastole, resistance to flow is decreased in the endocardium, resulting in greater flow to the endocardial layer. Eighty percent (80%) of LV coronary filling occurs during diastole. At a heart rate of 60 bpm, diastole occupies 2/3 of the cardiac cycle. As heart rate increases, the duration of diastole (SUPPLY) decreases as the relative length of systole (DEMAND) increases. Laver suggests an alternative hypothesis which focuses on the duration of recovery, rather than in increased oxygen demand.[2] He proposes that MVO_2 should be considered per beat (MVO_2/beat), rather than per unit of time (MVO_2/min). He supports this theory by citing data obtained during studies of pacing-induced tachycardia. Although minute MVO_2 increased, MVO_2/beat actually decreased! He concluded that tachycardia-induced angina pectoris resulted from incomplete time for recovery during each cardiac cycle; rather than an increase in MVO_2.

Maintenance of an adequate coronary perfusion pressure (CPP = diastolic BP - LV end diastolic pressure or PCWP) is important in patients with significant coronary artery disease. Normal coronary perfusion pressure = 60 mmHg. In patients with a stenotic or thrombosed coronary circulation, a greater CPP is necessary to maintain adequate perfusion beyond the site of obstruction.

It was initially thought that the amount of oxygen consumed was proportional to the amount of work the heart generates (Table 1). Subsequently, we have learned that the type of work the heart performs, influences MVO_2.[3] Increases in <u>flow work</u> (stroke volume) are associated with a smaller increase in MVO_2 than an equal amount of <u>pressure work</u>. The geometric basis for this observation is as follows:

LaPlace equation:	$P = T/r$	T = tension
For a sphere:	$T = Pr/2$	P = pressure
Volume of a sphere	$V = 4/3\ r^3$	r = radius
	$\therefore T = kPV^{0.33}$	K = constant

By substitution, LV wall tension is directly proportional to the pressure, but only to the cube root of the volume. Thus, increases in pressure create a greater wall tension and higher MVO_2 than does a similar change in volume.

A group of indirect indices of MVO_2 termed the rate pressure product (RPP) indices, are based on wall tension and heart rate. At present, the most widely used RPP term is heart rate x systolic blood pressure (RPP = HR x SBP). This index is based upon two hypotheses: 1) HR and SBP contribute equally to MVO_2 and 2) RPP correlates with MVO_2 over a wide range of HR and SBP. In man (awake state) RPP is a simple noninvasive calculation that has a reasonable correlation with the directly measured MVO_2.[4] Although RPP has been validated for the awake patient, analogous data does not exist for the anesthetized patient. One should consider these factors carefully when extrapolating data in awake patients to the supine anesthetized patient.[5] In exercise studies performed in the erect position, cardiac output and MVO_2 are increased as a result of increasing stroke volume. However, if exercise-induced stress is performed in the supine position, cardiac output is elevated mainly by an increase in heart rate rather than stroke volume. Further, changes in the contractile state of the heart, as seen with anesthetics, can greatly alter MVO_2, without changes in heart rate or blood pressure.

The differential effects of heart rate and systolic blood pressure have been evaluated in a canine model with fixed coronary stenosis.[6] RPP correlated poorly with directly measured MVO_2 and its value as a predictor of MVO_2 is invalid under many conditions. On the basis of myocardial lactate extraction, a given level of RPP could not be found that consistently predicted myocardial ischemia. As a matter of fact, no study exists that documents a good correlation between RPP and directly measured MVO_2 during general anesthesia.[7] The clinician who uses RPP for the anesthetized patient must be continuously aware of its limitations and should always consider the separate effects of HR and SBP on MVO_2. The fact that indirect indices, such as the RPP, are invalid for anesthetized patients, emphasizes the importance of alternative methods for detecting myocardial ischemia.

II. ISCHEMIA

Myocardial ischemia occurs when oxygen supply can no longer meet demand (Fig. 1). The ischemic state is associated with reduced perfusion (relative or absolute) and inadequate removal of metabolites. The heart extracts near maximal amounts of oxygen (arterial-coronary sinus O_2 difference). Thus, any increase in supply must be met by increases in coronary flow rather than extraction. Alterations either in coronary O_2 content or blood flow (global or regional) will affect coronary O_2 transport. Therefore, ischemia can result at varying myocardial metabolic requirements.

As a result of ischemia, a biochemical cascade is set into effect based on a switch from aerobic to anaerobic pathways. These biochemical changes are detectable within seconds of the ischemic event. Structural integrity of the myocardial cell is lost which implies the inability to actively transport Na+, K+, Mg++ and Ca++. Ischemia leading to cell death may be thought to occur in three phases: 1) loss of oxygen supply, 2) loss of metabolic substrate, and 3) inadequate removal of metabolites. With a loss of oxygen, adenosine triphosphate (ATP) levels are reduced. Consequently, decreased oxidative phosphorylation (oxidation of fatty acids to CO_2 and H_2O) results in abnormal diastolic relaxation and loss of contractile function (decreased ventricular compliance). During ischemia and acidosis which is associated with limited ATP production, ionic transport fails, synthesis of proteins and nucleic acids is reduced and a cellular autolytic process is begun with inadequate removal of cellular metabolites, these biochemical processes are amplified in the presence of poor perfusion . After these initial changes, a number of physiologic alterations occur which adversely effect left ventricular performance.

Ischemia results in decreased LV compliance.[8] Thus, the ventricle becomes "stiffer" and requires an increased filling pressure (PCWP) to maintain a given cardiac output. Subsequently ejection fraction decreases. If ischemia goes unrecognized, ventricular dilation and congestive heart failure occur. This is soon followed by cardiogenic shock and ultimately death. This emphasizes the role of early detection of myocardial ischemia, in that intervention may be performed at a stage of "reversible injury". Currently, the electrocardiogram forms the foundation for detection of ischemia. Inadequate interpretation of these critical cardiac events (inappropriate lead selection, inadequate calibration, unavailability of hard copy) may result in serious morbidity, or even mortality.

III. DIAGNOSIS OF ISCHEMIA IN THE ANESTHETIZED PATIENT

A. Is the patient the "best" monitor or myocardial infarction?

A notion exists that an "awake" patient, under a regional anesthetic (spinal or peridural), is a sensitive indicator of myocardial ischemia. Recent evidence suggests that this concept is incorrect and may lead to significant morbidity. A number of studies have documented the incidence of "silent ischemia" or asymptomatic coronary artery disease.[9] This entity can be defined as: the absence of angina (or its equivalents) in the presence of objective evidence of transient myocardial ischemia (EKG, radionuclear or echocardiographic studies, etc.). Three groups of patients may present with this disease process:

(a) Totally asymptomatic patients

(b) Asymptomatic patients post-myocardial infarction (MI) who have active ischemia

(c) Patients with angina who are asymptomatic with some ischemic episodes, but not with others.

At present, approximately two to four percent of asymptomatic males (greater than 45 years of age) and 20-30% of asymptomatic post MI patients have episodes of silent ischemia. The incidence of "silent" S-T segment depression (EKG) is quite high. More than 2/3 of ischemic events are undetected by "awake" patients. To further complicate matters, many of these events are not accompanied by significant alterations in heart rate or blood pressure. Slogoff and Keats have reported similar findings in a group of anesthetized patients undergoing coronary artery bypass surgery.[10] Only one third of these ischemic events were associated with hemodynamic abnormalities. A number of awake patients with silent ischemia have a "defective anginal warning system". It appears they have an altered perception of pain. On a theoretical basis, treatment with sedative or analgesic medications may further decrease their ability to perceive angina.

B. The electrocardiogram

The electrocardiogram (ECG) supplies an enormous amount of information regarding the status of the coronary circulation. By use a calibrated ECG (10 mm = 1 mV) employing leads V_5/II, 96% of EKG detectable ischemic events can be diagnosed.[11] ECG signs of ischemia include: ST segment change, alteration of the T wave and new onset of arrhythmias or conduction abnormalities, e.g., left bundle branch block (LBBB). The differential diagnosis of ST segment depression includes: left ventricular hypertrophy, digitalis effect and electrolyte alterations such as hypokalemia. However, electrocardiographic changes are usually a late sign of ischemia.[12] Clinically significant changes in ventricular compliance and regional wall motion precede the ECG alterations.[13] Consequently, at present, when ECG changes are observed, the clinician should be very therapeutically aggressive in limiting the extent and duration of ischemia.

C. Pulmonary artery monitoring

Since changes in ventricular compliance are among the earliest physiologic consequences of ischemia, the pulmonary artery catheter may also be useful in diagnosis. Kaplan and Wells reported that the presence of a prominent AC wave in PCWP tracing is consistent with myocardial ischemia.[14] Further, a fixed cardiac output with an increasing PCWP also suggests decreasing left ventricular compliance. Ischemia of the papillary muscle may lead to dilation of the LV and/or mitral valve apparatus. This may be detected by the presence of "v" waves in the PCWP trace.

D. Echocardiography

In the future, echocardiography or other non-invasive monitoring may help to detect early signs of ischemia, by discerning abnormalities in regional wall motion.[15] Regional wall motion can be assessed by using short axis (cross sectional) view. Qualitative analysis involves observing the moving 2-D tomographic cut for evidence of an abnormal contraction pattern during the cardiac cycle . An excellent agreement between electrocardiographic Q wave location and abnormally moving segments determined by 2-D echocardiography has been noted. Evidence suggests that wall motion abnormalities preceed ECG changes during ischemic episodes.[14] It is hoped that 2-D echocardiography will enable the clinician to detect ischemia earlier and institute therapy to prevent prolonged ischemic insult and infarction.

IV. TREATMENT STRATEGIES

Where possible, before initiating therapy, an attempt should be made to DIAGNOSE THE CAUSE OF ISCHEMIA. This will aid in choosing the appropriate pharmacologic therapy. Treatment pathways are suggested based on the major determinants of MVO_2. Various strategies are available to decrease demand or increase supply.

Decrease Demand	Increase supply
1. Vasodilators	1. O_2 content
2. Beta blockade	a. Hgb
3. Calcium channel blockers	b. F_IO_2
	2. Perfusion

Parenteral nitroglycerin (TNG) is the foundation of therapy for intraoperative myocardial ischemia. According to McGregor, nitroglycerin exerts it therapeutic effect by four possible mechanisms: 1) vasodilation of conduit vessels, 2) vasodilation of collateral vessels, 3) reduction in venous tone (preload) and 4) reduction of systolic blood pressure (afterload).[17,18]

Beta antagonists, such as propranolol, have played an important role in the management of ischemia. In addition to reducing heart rate and contractility, major determinants of MVO_2, propranolol also has membrane stabilizing effect ("quinidine-like"). Administration of propranolol (0.1 mg/kg) has been advocated for control of heart rate in the perioperative period. However, the use of beta blockade in a stressed patient may result in coronary vasoconstriction. Kern et al reported that a cold pressor test, (analogous to laryngoscopy and intubation) following propranolol pre-treatment (0.1 mg/kg) resulted in a 22% increase in coronary vasoconstriction.[19] Engel et al. also observed increases in coronary vascular tone in individuals who received propranolol prior to pacing induced tachycardia.[20] They also noted that the use of Calcium channel blockers in the same protocol improved coronary perfusion.

On this basis, calcium channel blockers, such as verapamil, may offer a significant therapeutic advantage. In a manner similar to beta blockers, MVO_2 is reduced (negative inotropic and negative chronotropic effects). More important, myocardial oxygen supply is improved by increasing perfusion (decreased coronary vascular resistance). In this regard, coronary vasospastic decrease (Prinzmetal's angina) may be exacerbated by beta blockers. Consequently, when the diagnosis of coronary spasm is entertained (elevated ST-segment), calcium channel blockers and nitrates should be administered.

Although it is difficult to set an arbitrary level of heart rate for decisions regarding initiation of therapy, clinically I find a heart rate = 80 bpm a useful starting point useful. Knowledge of blood pressure (BP), cardiac output (CO) and pulmonary capillary wedge pressure (PCWP) complete the hemodynamic picture upon which to guide therapy (Fig. 2).

A. Treatment Algorithm

1. Heart rate 60-80 bpm

If signs of ischemia occur with a low heart rates (60-80 bpm), nitroglycerin is preferable therapy. Adsorption through plastics, (plastic containers, PVC intravenous tubing or cardiopulmonary bypass apparatus) results in a significant loss of nitroglycerin.[21] Therefore, nitroglycerin should be delivered from glass containers through special non-absorbing tubing. Intravascular volume status should be restored or severe hypotension may occur. In studies we conducted, it appears that the efficacy of nitroglycerin as a vasodilator in the anesthetized patient (narcotic) is seen at doses less than 3 ug/kg/min.[22] In a patient with a critical coronary obstruction, a relatively small increase in heart rate from 65 to 75 bpm may provoke an ischemic episode. In this subset, the addition of beta blockers or calcium channel blockers are useful.

2. Heart rate greater than 90 bpm

At heart rates greater than 90 bpm, therapy should be directed at reducing heart rate. The beta blocker propranolol is a first line drug. Intravenous propranolol can be administered in doses of 0.1-0.25 mg/increment up to a total dose of 0.10 mg/kg (7 mg in a 70 kg individual). Propranolol may adversely affect left ventricular performance. It is important to have measurements of LV filling pressure (PCWP) and cardiac output. If PCWP increases, and cardiac output decreases, propranolol therapy should be discontinued. As mentioned previously, calcium channel blockers may have certain therapeutic benefits when compared to propranolol in this situation.[19,22] Specifically, the calcium channel blockers increase myocardial O_2 supply, while propranolol decreases myocardial demand. Verapamil, the only parenteral calcium channel blocker available in the United States is administered in 1.25-2.50 mg increments to a dose of approximately 5-10 mg. Low dose nitroglycerin (3 ug/Kg/min) infusion is also given to achieve the associated therapeutic benefit.

Tachycardia (on the basis of a hyperdynamic state) associated with increased blood pressure, cardiac output, with a normal or increased left ventricular filling pressure, may indicate a need for additional depth of anesthesia. Vasodilator therapy is initiated if clinically the patient is thought to have an adequate level of anesthesia. If ischemia and tachycardia are still present, beta blockers may be added.

TACHYCARDIA IS AN APPROPRIATE PHYSIOLOGIC RESPONSE TO HYPOVOLEMIA AND/OR ANEMIA. Therefore, it is imperative before embarking on major cardiovascular therapy to assure yourself that the patient has adequate left ventricular filling pressures (PCWP = 10 mmHg).

If ischemia results in cardiac failure (BP PCWP CO), a combination of preload reduction (vasodilator therapy-nitroglycerin) and inotropic support (e.g. dobutamine) may be beneficial. An increase in the inotropic state can result in higher myocardial oxygen demands. However, by reducing ventricular diameter and wall stress, augmentation of inotropic state may actually reduce myocardial oxygen demand; since ventricular diameter is reduced.

3. Heart Rate Less Than 60 bpm

Finally, ischemia associated with bradycardia may be treated with TNG and/or atropine. If a muscle relaxant is required, pancuronium may be an excellent choice in this clinical setting.

Summary

Early recognition of myocardial ischemia by currently available methods can be difficult. However, the anesthesiologist still can detect myocardial ischemia, by invasive, non-invasive methods. When it is recognized, early and aggressive therapy is mandated to prevent circulatory consequences, including congestive heart failure, cardiogenic shock, and death.

References

1. Slogoff S, Keats AS: Does perioperative myocardial ischemia lead to postoperative myocardial infarction? Anesthesiology 62:107-114, 1985.
2. Laver MB: Myocardial ischaemia: Dilemma between information available and information demand. Br Heart J 50:222-230, 1983.
3. Sarnoff SJ, Braunwald E, Welch GH Jr, et al: Hemodynamic determinants of oxygen consumption of the heart with special reference to the tension-time index. Am J Physiol 192:148-156, 1958.

4. Kitamura K, Jorgensen CR, Gobel FL, et al.: Hemodynamic correlates of myocardial oxygen consumption during upright exercise. J Appl Physiol 32:516-522, 1972.
5. Barash PG, and Kopriva C: Editorial: The Rate Pressure Product in Clinical Anesthesia -- Boon or Bane? Anesth & Analg 59:229-231, 1980.
6. Barash PG, Seinfeld F, Kay H, Condos S, Hashim S, Tinker J, Geha AS: RPP: May it R.I.P. Anesthesiology 57:A22, 1982.
7. Moffitt EA, Sethna DH, Gray RJ, et al.: Rate pressure produce correlates poorly with myocardial oxygen consumption during anaesthesia in coronary patients. Can Anaesth Soc J 31:5-12, 1984.
8. Gaasch WH, Levine HJ, Quinones MA, Alexander JK: Left ventricular compliance: Mechanisms and clinical implications. Am J Cardiol 38:645-653, 1976.
9. Cohn PF: Silent myocardial ischemia: Present status. Mod Concepts Cardiovasc Dis 56:1-5, 1987.
10. Slogoff S, Keats AS. Further observations on perioperative myocardial ischemia. Anesthesiology 65:539-542, 1986.
11. Blackburn H, Katigbak R: What ECG leads to take after exercise. Am Heart J 67:184-185, 1964.
12. Scheuer J, Brachfeld N: Coronary insufficiency: relations between hemodynamic, electrical, and biochemical parameters. Circ Res 18:178-189, 1966.
13. Upton MT, Rerych SK, Newman GE, Port S, Cobb FR, Jones RH: Detecting abnormalities in left ventricular function during exercise before angina and ST-segment depression. Circulation 62:341-349, 1980.
14. Kaplan JA, Wells PH: Early diagnosis of myocardial ischemia using the pulmonary arterial catheter. Anesth Analg 60:789-793, 1981.
15. LaMantia KR, Lehmann KG, Barash PG: Echocardiography in the Perioperative Period. Acute Care (In Press)
16. Battler A, Froelicher VF, Gallagher KP, Kemper P, et al.: Dissociation between regional myocardial dysfunction and ECG changes during ischemia in the conscious dog. Circulation 62:735-744, 1980.
17. McGregor M: The nitrates and myocardial ischemia (Editorial). Circulation 66:689-692, 1982.
18. Feldman RL, Conti CR: Editorial: Relief of myocardial ischemia with nitroglycerin: What is the mechanism? 64:1098-1100, 1981

19. Kern MJ, Ganz P, Horowitz JD, et al.: Potentiation of coronary vasoconstriction by beta-adrenergic blockade in patients with coronary artery disease. Circulation 67:1178-1184, 1983.
20. Engel HJ, Lichtlen PR: Beneficial enhancement of coronary blood flow by nifedipine. Am J Med 71:658-666, 1981.
21. Cote DD, Torchia MG: Nitroglycerin adsorption to polyvinylchloride seriously interferes with its clinical use. Anesth Analg 55:541-543, 1982.
22. Braunwald E: Mechanism of action of calcium-channel blocking agents. N Engl J Med 307:1618-1627, 1982.

TABLE I

Determinants of Myocardial Oxygen Consumption (MVO_2) - Normal Beating Heart

	Contribution to MVO_2 %
MAJOR	
Myocardial tension development	30-40
Heart rate	--*
Contractile state	10-15
MINOR	
External work	10-15
Basal metabolism	25
Electrical/chemical activity	1

* Determines cumulative active energy expenditure per minute.

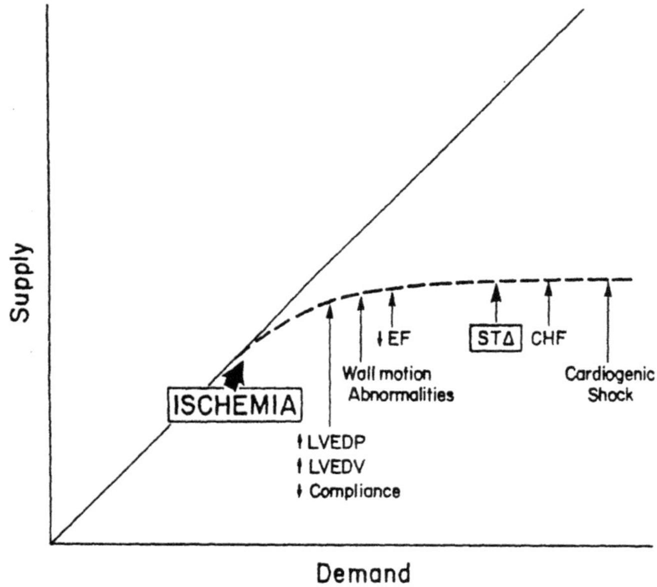

Figure 1: Hemodynamic consequences of myocardial ischemia. Ischemia occurs when demand exceeds supply. (LVEDP = left ventricular diastolic pressure; LVEDV = left ventricular end diastolic volume; EF = ejection fraction; ST = ST segment change; CHF = congestive heart failure)

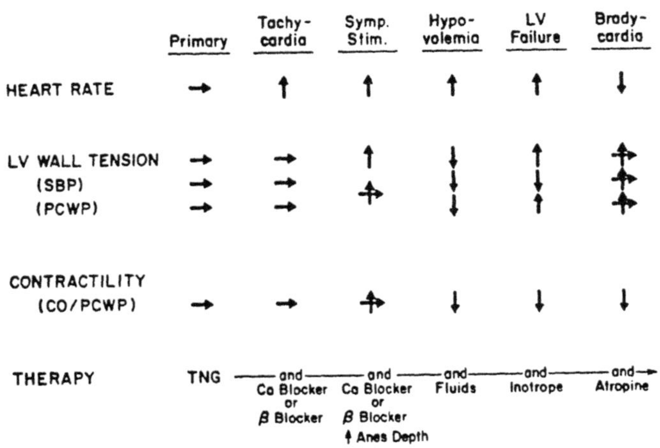

Figure 2: Protocol for treatment of myocardial ischemia.

THE RIGHT VENTRICLE : FORGOTTEN TOO LONG !

P. FOËX , C.ARVIEUX and J.G. RAMSAY

Introduction

Experimental evidence in which extensive destruction of the free wall of the right ventricle did not cause a significant increase in central venous pressure (1) or a marked reduction in cardiac output (2), has led to the view that right ventricular contraction may not be important for the maintenance of an adequate circulatory function.

However, relatively recently, Laver recognized (3) that acute right ventricular dysfunction occurs in critically ill patients and is an important determinant of the overall effect of acute illnesses, especially respiratory failure, on the circulation. Marked abnormalities in cardiovascular function have been identified in patients with respiratory failure. These include pulmonary arterial hypertension, elevated pulmonary vascular resistance and depressed right and left ventricular performance. Intermittent positive pressure ventilation, particularly when associated with positive end-expiratory pressure improves arterial oxygenation but may exert adverse effects on the cardiovascular system.

The right ventricle

Because of contrasting functional demands, the human heart is not a simple pair of parallel pumps, despite the fact that the right and left ventricles deliver the same amount of blood. The right ventricle is a crescent shaped, thin walled cavity bordered by a concave free wall and the convex interventricular septum. The right ventricle possesses an inflow orifice (the tricuspid valve), an inflow tract leading at an obtuse angle to an outflow tract (the infundibulum), and an outflow orifice (the pulmonary valve). The infundibulum may provide support for the pulmonary valve cusps by maintaining some of its contractile tone during diastole. The outflow tract of the right ventricle is anatomically and embryologically different from the main portion of the right ventricle.

The myocardium of the right ventricle consists of fibres within a network of supportive connective tissue. The direction of imbrication of fibres reverses at the equator in a figure of eight. The attachment of the right ventricular free wall to the left ventricular and septal myocardium contributes to the inter-dependence between the ventricles and facilitates right ventricular emptying, (4,5). The extreme complexity of the fibre paths explains the complex nature of right ventricular contraction, the differences in regional patterns of contraction, and the interactions between right and left ventricles.

Interactions between right and left ventricles

a) Muscle: As some fibres pathways run continuously from the free wall of the right ventricle to the septum and the anterior wall of the left ventricle, there is mechanical linkage of the ventricles and, therefore, changes in the dimensions and performance of one ventricle influence the geometry of the other.

b) Septum: A radial force is created by the tethering action of the muscle fibres and dominates in the direction of the free wall of the left ventricle. Axial forces are a function of the chamber pressure and the surface area of the septum and tend to bow the septum toward the right ventricle (6).

Under normal conditions axial forces dominate on the left ventricular surface of the septum so that it bowes into the right ventricle throughout the cardiac cycle. However, acute or chronic increases in right ventricular pressure or volume alter the distribution of axial forces causing a shift of the septum towards the left ventricle (3,7). Thus, the geometry and distensibility of the left ventricle are modified by changes in right ventricular dynamics and vice-versa.

c) Pericardium: Pressure coupling between the ventricles is tight when the pericardium is closed (8,9) and the heart is best viewed as a composite pericardium - myocardium shell. In this shell, the ventricular muscle is more elastic than the pericardium (10).

d) Intrathoracic pressure: Negative pressure during inspiration increases the gradient between extra and intrathoracic veins; this facilitates the filling of the right heart. However, venous return to the left ventricle is not facilitated because the filling reservoir of the left ventricle (i.e the pulmonary vascular bed) is subjected to the intrathoracic pressure as much as the ventricle itself (11).

With intermittent positive pressure ventilation, mean intrathoracic pressure increases, particularly when positive end-expiratory pressure is used. This is accompanied by an increase in the radius of curvature of the septum (8).

Determinants of right ventricular performance

Afterload. The marked influence of afterload on the right ventricular stroke volume has been demonstrated by Ghignone, Girling and Previtt (12). Increases in pulmonary vascular resistance by pulmonary artery embolisation were shown to cause marked reductions of stroke volume. Because of its thin wall, the right ventricle, is more sensitive to an increase in afterload than the left ventricle.

Preload and contractility. In elegant studies of right ventricular pump function, Weber and his colleagues (13) have examined the relationship between stroke volume and ejection pressure. They showed that an increase in preload, represented by an increase in end-diastolic volume, shifts the right ventricular pump function curve upwards and to the right. They also showed that dopamine, at constant end-diastolic volume, causes a significant improvement of right ventricular pump function thus demonstrating that changes in inotropy influence right ventricular performance.

Compliance. The right ventricular compliance is substantially greater than the left ventricular compliance. However, because of the pericardium, right ventricular compliance is influenced by the filling pressure of the left ventricle. Increases in left ventricular end-diastolic pressure reduce, while reductions in left ventricular end-diastolic pressure increase, right ventricular compliance. This interaction is caused by changes in the radius of curvature of the interventricular septum (6,7). Similarly, increases in right ventricular filling modify left ventricular compliance. In many patients suffering from the adult respiratory distress syndrome, the pulmonary capillary wedge pressure is elevated even though the end-diastolic volume of the left ventricle is not increased. This indicates that right ventricular dilatation (due to pulmonary hypertension) decreases left ventricular compliance (6). Pharmacologically mediated reductions in pulmonary vascular resistance unload the right ventricle and by this mechanism increase left ventricular compliance, presumably by reducing the degree of leftward shift of the septum.

Patterns of right ventricular contraction

Contraction begins with the downward motion of the tricuspid valve, followed by the inward motion of the free wall. Finally, an inward motion of the septum contributes to right ventricular ejection.

Asynchrony of regional contraction.

The development of methods of assessing regional ventricular function has revealed that contraction of the free wall of the right ventricle is neither uniform nor synchronous (Fig.1).

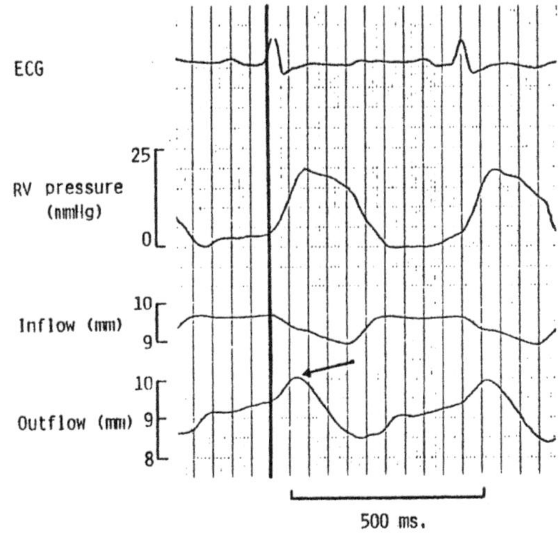

Figure 1. Simultaneous recordings of ECG, right ventricular pressure, inflow tract and outflow tract wall motion (sonomicrometry), showing that the onset of shortening (downward deflection) occurs later in the outflow tract (arrow) than in the inflow tract.

Contraction starts in the inflow tract and progresses toward the outflow tract in a peristalsis-like fashion. Outflow tract contraction lags behind inflow tract contraction by at least 25 milliseconds (14). This delay in onset of contraction is caused by a delay in electrical activation (15). In the early phase of systole, the inflow tract contracts while the outflow tract dilates. Shortening in the outflow tract persists during a substantial portion of diastole. It has been postulated that the outflow tract, under resting conditions, acts as a buffer to protect the pulmonary vasculature. However, when the right ventricle is stimulated the delay between outflow and inflow tract contraction becomes shorter and right ventricular contraction becomes more synchronous (14).

The regional differences in right ventricular contraction and relaxation are enhanced by interventions such as positive end-expiratory pressure (PEEP) and pulmonary hypertension. The application of PEEP (up to 20 cm H_2O) has relatively little effect on the end-diastolic pressure-dimension relationship of the outflow tract (Fig.2) while it causes profound changes in the inflow tract where dimensions are decreased and compliance is reduced significantly (16). Similarly, outflow tract shortening, irrespective of the filling pressure of the right ventricle, is hardly influenced by PEEP, while inflow tract shortening, at low and mid-range filling pressures, is profoundly reduced.

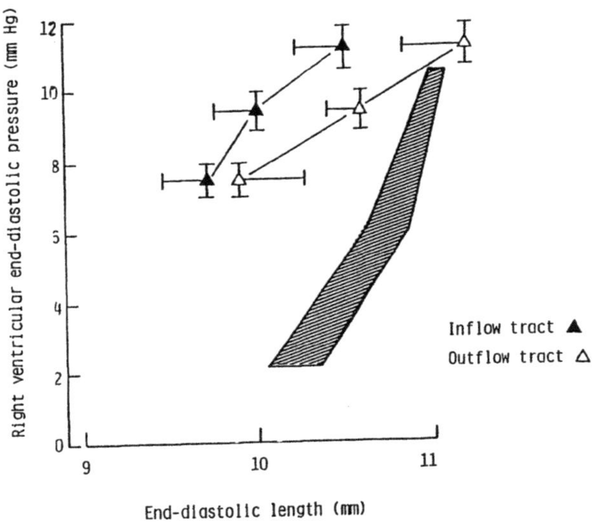

Figure 2. In the dog, the relationship between right ventricular end-diastolic pressure and dimensions is shifted upwards and to the left by positive end-expiratory pressure (PEEP 20 cmH_2O). The shift is greater for the inflow tract (open symbols) than for the outflow tract (closed symbols). The shaded area represents the pressure-dimensions of both the inflow and outflow tracts before administration of PEEP (after Watkins et al,1985 [17]).

Coronary blood flow

While coronary blood flow to the left ventricle occurs predominantly during diastole, coronary blood flow to the right ventricle occurs during both systole and diastole. Kolin, Gaal and Austin (18) have shown that left coronary flow is essentially diastolic, while right coronary flow occurs predominantly during ventricular systole. This is not surprising since the "coronary driving pressure" (the difference between aortic pressure and right ventricular pressure) is high throughout the cardiac cycle. However, in the presence of pulmonary hypertension, right ventricular pressure increases and systolic coronary flow is maintained only as long as aortic pressure is high (19). It is now recognised that an adequate aortic pressure is essential if right ventricular function is to be maintained in the face of pulmonary hypertension. If this requirement is not met, right ventricular coronary flow will be insufficient to supply enough oxygen to the wall of the right ventricle and the right ventricle will fail. In these circumstances, peripheral vasoconstriction restores the coronary driving pressure and improves cardiac output (20).

During experiments involving pulmonary artery banding, a linear relationship has been observed between both stroke volume or inflow tract shortening and right ventricular coronary perfusion pressure (Fig.3). The administration of phenylephrine caused peripheral vasoconstriction thus restoring the pressure gradient between aorta and right ventricle. This, in turn, increased right ventricular coronary blood flow and improved both inflow tract shortening and stroke volume. Similarly, in patients suffering from right ventricular failure due to severe pulmonary hypertension, and associated with systemic hypotension, noradrenaline can be successfully used to improve right ventricular myocardial perfusion and cardiac output.

The effects of PEEP in the presence of pulmonary hypertension have not been extensively studied. However, experiments involving pulmonary banding suggest that moderate levels of PEEP (7.5 cm H_2O) may cause significant worsening of cardiac performance. In patients with right ventricular failure, PEEP may cause exaggerated circulatory impairment.

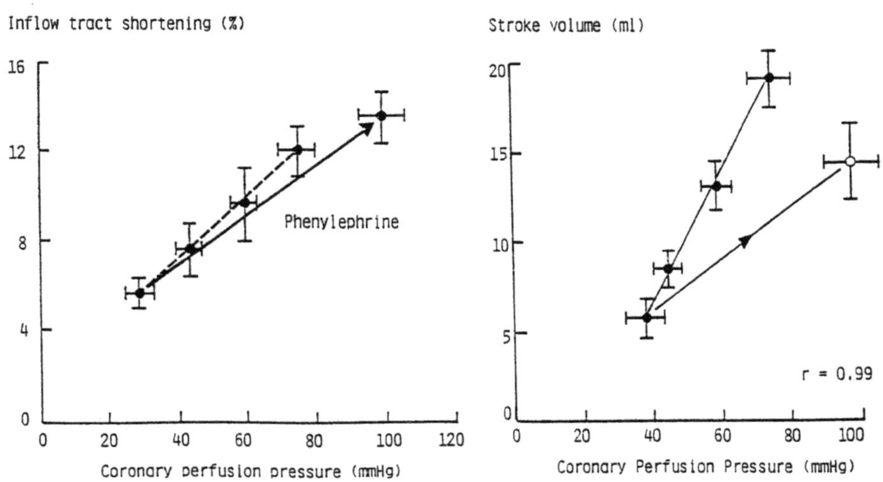

Figure 3. In anaesthetized dogs, subjected to gradual pulmonary artery banding, linear relationships have been observed between inflow tract shortening and right coronary artery perfusion pressure (left hand panel) and between stroke volume and coronary perfusion pressure (right hand panel). Phenylephrine brings about a substantial increase in coronary perfusion pressure, inflow tract shortening and stroke volume.

While failure of the circulation due primarily to right ventricular failure is not very commonon, it is important to recognise its existance and to prevent the development of systemic hypotension, because the latter will have a detrimental effect on right ventricular perfusion. Thus far attempts at reducing pulmonary hypertension with vasodilators, especially prostacyclin, have been successful only when systemic arterial pressure was maintained by the simultaneous administration of vasospressors (20). Before considering complex interventions such as pulmonary artery balloon counter pulsation (21) or right ventricular assist devices (22) attempts should be made at improving right ventricular perfusion with vasoconstrictors.

References

1 Starr, I., Jeffers, W.A. and Meade, J.R. (1943). The absence of conspicuous increments of venous pressure after severe damage to the right ventricle of the dog, with a discussion of the relation between clinical congestive failure and heart disease. Am.Heart J., **26**, 291-301.

2 Brooks, H., Kirk, E.S., Vokonas, P.S., Urschel, C.W. and Sonnenblick, E.H. (1971). Performance of the right ventricle under stress: relation to right coronary flow. J.Clin.Invest., **50**, 2176-2183.

3 Laver, M.B., Strauss, H.W., and Pohost, G.M. (1979). Right and left ventricular geometry: adjustments during acute respiratory failure. Crit.Care Med., **7**, 509-519.

4 Streeter,D.D.jr., Vaishnav,R.V., Patel,D.J., Spotniz,H.M., Ross,J.jr., and Sonnenblick E.H. (1970). Stress distribution in the canine left ventricle during diastole and systole. Biophys.J.,**10**, 345-363.

5 McCallum,J.B. (1900). On the muscular architecture and growth of the ventricles of the heart. Welch Festschrift. Johns Hopkins Hosp.Reports.,**9**, 307-335.

6 Weber, K.T., Janicki, J.S., Shroff, S.G., Likoff, M.J., St.John Sutton, M.G. (1983). The right ventricle: Physiologic and pathophysiologic considerations. Crit.Care Med., **11**, 323-328.

7 Jardin, F., Eveleigh, M.C., Gurdjian, F., Delille, F. and Margairaz, A. (1979). Venous admixture in human septic shock; comparative effects of blood volume expansion, dopamine infusion and isoprotenerol infusion on mismatching of ventilation and pulmonary blood flow in peritonitis. Circulation, **60**, 155-159.

8 Laks, M.M., Garner,D., and Swan, H.J.C. (1967) Volumes and compliance measured simultaneously in the right and left ventricles of the dog. Circulation Res.,**20**, 565-569.

9 Elzinga,G., Von Grondelle, R., Westerof,N., and van den Bos,G.C.(1974) Ventricular interference. Am.J.Physiol.,**226**, 941-947.

10 Glantz,S.A., Misbach,G.A., Moores,W.Y., Mathey, D.G., Lekven,J., Stowe,D.F., Parmley,W.W., and Tyberg,J.V. (1978) The pericardium substantially affects the left ventricular diastolic pressure - volume relationship in the dog. Circ.Res.,**42**, 433-441

11 Weber,K.T., Janicki,J.S., Shroff,S.G., and Likoff, M.J. (1983). The cardiopulmonary unit. The body's gas transport system. Clin.Chest Med.,**4,(2)**, 101-110.

12 Ghignone, M., Girling, L. and Prewitt, R.M. (1984) Effect of increased pulmonary vascular resistance on right ventricular systolic performance in dogs. Am.J.Physiol., **246**, H339-H343.

13 Weber, K.T., Janicki, J.S., Shroff, S. and Fishman, A.P. (1981). Contractile mechanics and interaction of the right and left ventricles. Am.J.Cardiol.,**47**, 686-695.

14 Raines, R.A., LeWinter, M.M. and Covell, J.W. (1976). Regional shortening patterns in canine right ventricle. Am.J.Physiol. **231**, 1395-1400.

15 Freud, G.E., Stern, M.C., Watson, H. and Durrer, D. (1975). Activation of the hypertrophic right ventricle in the dog. Cardiovasc.Res., **9**, 302-313.

16 Meier, G.D., Bove, A.A., Santamore, W.P. and Lynch, P.R. (1980). Contractile function in canine right ventricle. Am.J.Physiol., **239**, H794-H804.

17 Watkins,J.,Foëx,P.,Stone,J.G. and LeWinter,M.M.(1984) Effect of PEEP on regional right ventricular function. Circulation,**70**,Suppl II,II-181.

18 Kolin, A., Ross,G., Gaal, P. and Austin, S. (1964). Simultaneous electromagnetic measurements of blood flow in the major coronary arteries. Nature (Lond.), **203**, 148-150.

19 Vlahakes, G.J., Turley, K., and Hoffman, J.I.E. (1981). The pathophysiology of failure in acute right ventricular hypertension: hemodynamic and biochemical correlations. Circulation, **63**, 87-95.

20 Symbas,P.N., McKeown,P.P., Santora,A.H., and Vlasis,S.E.(1985). Pulmonary artery balloon counterpulsation for treatment of intraoperative right ventricular failure. Ann.Thor.Surg.,**39**, 437-440.

21 D'Ambra,M.N., LaRaia,P.J., Philbin,D.M., Watkins,W.D., Hilgenberg,A.D., and Buckley,M.J.(1985). Prostaglandins E_1. A new therapy for refractory right heart failure and pulmonary hypertension after mitral valve replacement. J.Thorac.Cardiovasc.Surg.,**89**, 567-572.

22 Pennington,D.G., Merjavy,J.P., Swartz,M.T., Codd,J.E., Barner,H.B., Lagunoff, D., Bashiti,H., Kaiser,G.C., and Willman,V.L.(1985). The importance of biventricular failure in patients with postoperative cardiogenic shock. Ann.Thor.Surg., **39**, 16-24.

UPDATE ON INTERACTIONS BETWEEN CALCIUM ANTAGONISTS AND ANESTHETICS

R. MERIN

The cardiovascular effects of the potent inhalation anesthetics, halothane, enflurane and isoflurane[1] are remarkably similar to those produced by the calcium antagonist drugs, verapamil, diltiazem and nifedipine.[5-7] Bosnjak et al have even shown similar effects on sino-atrial node conduction[8] and calcium entry in heart muscle.[9] Lynch and co-workers have also indicated that the inhalation anesthetics have electrophysiologic effects in heart muscle which suggest interference in calcium entry.[10-12] It is of some interest that the cardioactive calcium antagonists, verapamil and diltiazem, appear to superficially resemble halothane and enflurane in that they produce more cardiac depression whereas the dihydroperidines such as nifedipine and nicardipine appear to resemble isoflurane, producing more peripheral vasodilation.

Nevertheless, many of the studies, both in animals and man, have indicated that the two classes of drugs when given in clinical concentrations or doses produce minimal cardiovascular interaction.[13-25] Nevertheless, there have been some reports of marked cardiovascular depression produced by the combination of potent inhalation anesthetics and the calcium antagonist.[26-29] When the two groups of studies are compared, however, there is a common thread. All of the studies which show marked interaction between the calcium antagonist and the inhalation anesthetics are in open chest animals. The effects of either drug individually in this preparation are considerably greater than those seen in closed chest animals. For instance, in the study by Priebe and Skarvan, isoflurane administered to dogs basally anesthetized with fentanyl-droperidol and given an infusion of diltiazem produced marked dose-related depressant effects on all aspects of ventricular function both right and left.[28] In a slightly different protocol, Kapur and co-workers have looked at the effect of increasing plasma levels of diltiazem during steady state low concentrations (1+ MAC isoflurane).[15] Plasma levels equivalent to those documented by Priebe and Skarvan produced minimal effects on ventricular function with only slight depression of left ventricular dP/dt and elevation of pulmonary artery occluded pressures being seen. Of particular note, there was no change in heart rate, mean aortic pressure or cardiac index. Using a left heart bypass preparation in the dog, Kates et al showed marked depression of ventricular function by very low plasma concentrations of verapamil (less than 50 $ng \cdot ml^{-1}$) and subanesthetic concentrations of isoflurane (0.5%).[26] Videcoq et al studied the effect of one low dose of verapamil (250 $\mu g \cdot kg^{1}$ given over 30 minutes, followed by an infusion of 60 μg/kg/hr) producing mean plasma verapamil levels between 45 and 50 $ng \cdot ml^{-1}$ during subanesthetic concentrations of isoflurane (1% inspired).[29] They observed a 20% decrease in stroke volume and a 15% decrease in cardiac output and equivalent depression in aortic blood flow acceleration, left ventricular peak power and dP/dt max. Studies by Kapur and co-workers[14] and Rogers et al[17] showed minimal effects on ventricular function and considerably higher isoflurane and verapamil doses in closed chest animals. Another open chest preparation looked at the interaction between halothane (1% inspired) and verapamil without measured plasma verapamil levels.[27] Low dose verapamil (320 $\mu g \cdot kg^{-1}$ cumulative over a period of 60 min) produced marked depression of ventricular function with significant increases in left ventricular end-diastolic pressure and end-diastolic fiber length and a 38% decrease in stroke volume, 32% decrease in cardiac output, 39% decrease in left ventricular dP/dt, and a 50% decrease in peak aortic blood flow acceleration. At comparable halothane concentrations and probable verapamil plasma levels (which they measured and Ramsay et al did not), Kapur et al[14] and Chelly et al[16] both saw minimal effects of the combination of halothane and verapamil on hemodynamic performance. The only open chest preparation which failed to show marked cardiovascular depressant interaction between a calcium antagonist and an inhalation anesthetic was that of Tosone et al.[30] A bolus dose of nifedipine, even given during 2% halothane, produced minimal hemodynamic effects, suggesting that the dihydroperidine calcium blockers may be better tolerated even by the open chest animal. Another dihydroperidine calcium blocker, nicardipine, also produced only vasodilation and arterial hypotension even during deep isoflurane anesthesia in the chronically instrumented closed chest dog.[18] In closed chest animals, including swine[31] and dogs in both acute[14,15,20,32] and chronic models[16-19], only with high doses of anesthetics (greater than 1.5 mac) and/or high plasma levels of the calcium blockers were clinically significant hemodynamic interactions observed. In fact, the major detrimental interaction in both the acute and chronic studies was related to severely depressed atrioventricular conduction and sinus arrest which resulted in severe bradycardia (less than 30 min^{-1}) which was resistant to treatment unless the inhalation anesthetics have been discontinued. The studies in humans conducted with low dose calcium blockers and low concentrations of anesthetics[21-25] also showed minimal hemodynamic interaction. On the other hand, all experiments conducted in open chest, heavily instrumented animals have shown marked depression of ventricular function produced by the interaction of both diltiazem and verapamil and halothane and isoflurane.

In retrospect, these observations are predictable. It has been shown that verapamil is much more depressant to ventricular function in patients whose ventricular function is already compromised by disease.[33] Consequently, it would be expected that high concentrations of inhalation anesthetics, which do depress ventricular function, would produce more interaction with even low concentrations of the cardioactive calcium blocking drugs. It has also been well demonstrated that the open chest, instrumented animal is a very different physiologic preparation than even acutely anesthetized, closed chest animals and certainly than chronically instrumented, closed chest animals.[34,35] The fact that subtherapeutic concentrations of verapamil and subanesthetic concentrations of isoflurane produce such marked hemodynamic depression[7,10,11] is graphic demonstration of this observation.

Although the calcium channel blocking drugs may be of some use given intravenously during anesthesia, the more common clinical problem is the management of patients who have been chronically treated with these drugs. It is probably not warranted to extrapolate interactions from intravenously administered calcium blockers, even with steady state plasma levels, to patients chronically treated with oral drugs. Bonow and co-workers have shown that the effect of intravenous versus chronic verapamil is different in patients with hypertrophic cardiomyopathies.[36] Our laboratory has recently studied the effect of chronically administered verapamil and the three inhalation anesthetics, and have found that even at higher plasma verapamil levels than those measured in our acute experiments the hemodynamic effects of the inhalation anesthetics were quantitatively less.[19] In addition, Kapur and co-workers have shown that patients treated with a combination of beta blockers and nifedipine tolerated high dose fentanyl anesthesia for coronary artery revascularization without difficulty and even showed no undue depression of ventricular function when verapamil was infused intravenously during anesthesia.[25] Finally, patients taking calcium channel blockers preoperatively were not observed to have any conduction block in the perioperative period even when concurrent beta adrenergic blocking drugs were also been taken.[37]

In addition to the pharmacodynamic interactions between calcium antagonists and anesthetics referred to above, there also are significant pharmacokinetic interactions. Chelly et al have shown in chronically instrumented dogs that all three inhalation anesthetics (halothane, enflurane and isoflurane) produce a significant decrease in intercompartmental clearance, initial and steady-state volume of distribution, and total clearance of intravenously administered verapamil. Likewise, isoflurane also decreases the initial and steady-state volume of distribution and total clearance of the dihydroperidine calcium antagonist, nicardipine.[39] Since both steady-state volume of distribution and total clearance were equally depressed, there was no change in the elimination half-life produced by the inhalation anesthetics. However, intravenous administration of the same dose of either verapamil or the dihydroperidines to patients awake and anesthetized with these anesthetics will produce much higher plasma levels in the anesthetized patients. Obviously, this has important clinical implications. The mechanism of these pharmacokinetic effects is less clear. Certainly since the calcium antagonists are cleared predominantly by the liver, any effects on liver blood flow and/or extraction would be expected to markedly affect their metabolism. Certainly there is evidence to suggest that both halothane and enflurane significantly decrease liver blood flow in clinical concentrations.[41,42] However, no such effect has been shown for isoflurane.[17] On the other hand, there is evidence that depression of cardiac output can result in decreased volume of distribution of high hepatic clearance drugs (lidocaine).[43] In addition, the fact that verapamil's intercompartmental clearance was decreased by the inhalation anesthetics suggests that redistribution of blood flow during exposure to volatile anesthetics may be important in the pharmacokinetic properties. These mechanisms need further exploration.

REFERENCES

1. Merin, R.G. Surg. Clin. N. Amer. 55:769-773, 1975.
2. Merin, R.G., Kumazawa, T., Luka, N.L. Anesthesiology 44:401-413, 1976.
3. Merin, R.G., Kumazawa, T., Luka, N.L. Anesthesiology 45:501-507, 1976.
4. Merin, R.G., Basch, S. Anesthesiology 55:398-408, 1981.
5. Henry, P.D. Am. J. Cardiol. 46:1047-1057, 1980.
6. Walsh, R.A., et al: Am. Heart J. 102:341-350, 1981.
7. Bongrani, S., et al. J. Cardiovasc. Pharmacol. 7:899-905, 1985.
8. Bosnjak, Z.J., Kampine, J.P. Anesthesiology 58:314-321, 1983.
9. Bosnjak, Z.J., Kampine, J.P. Am. J. Physiol. 251:H374-381, 1986.
10. Lynch, C., Vogel, M., Sperelakis, N. Anesthesiology 55:360-368, 1981.
11. Lynch, C., Vogel, S., Pratila, M.D., Sperelakis, N. J. Pharmacol. Exp. Ther. 222:405-409, 1982.
12. Lynch, C. Anesthesiology 64:620-631, 1986.
13. Kapur, P.A., Flacke, W.E. Anesthesiology 55:218-225, 1981.
14. Kapur, P.A., Bloor, B.C., Flacke, W.E., Olewine, S.K. Anesthesiology 61:156-160, 1984.
15. Kapur, P.A., Campos, J.H., Tippit, S.E. Anesth. Analg. 65:81-87, 1986.
16. Chelly, J.E., Rogers, K., Hysing, E.S., Taylor, A., Hartley, C., Merin, R.G. Anesthesiology 64:560-567, 1986.
17. Rogers, K., Hysing, E.S., Merin, R.G., Taylor, A., Hartley, C., Chelly, J.E. Anesthesiology 64:568-575, 1986.
18. Hysing. E., Chelly, J.E., Doursout, M-F., Hartley, C., Merin, R.G. Anesthesiology 65:385-391, 1986.
19. Merin, R.G., Chelly, J.E., Hysing, E.S., Rogers, K., Dlewati, A., Hartley, C.J., Abernethy, D.R., Doursout, M-F. Anesthesiology 66:140-146, 1987.
20. Kapur, P.A., Matarazzo, D.A., Fung, D.M., Sullivan, K.B. Anesthesiology 66:122-129, 1987.

21. Kates, R.A., Kaplan, J.A. Anesth. Analg. 62:821-826, 1983.
22. Schulte-Sasse, U., Hess, W., Markschies-Hornung, A., Tarnow, J. Thorac. Cardiovasc. Surg. 31:261-265, 1983.
23. Schulte-Sasse, U., Hess, W., Markschies-Hornung, A., Tarnow, J. Anesth. Analg. 63:791-798, 1984.
24. Kishi. Y., Okumura, F., Furuya, H. Br. J. Anaesth. 56:1003-1007, 1984.
25. Kapur, P.A., Norel, E.J., Dajee, H., Cohen, G., Flacke, W. Can. Anaesth. Soc. J. 33:138-144, 1986.
26. Kates, R.A., Kaplan, J.A., Guyton, R.A., Dorsey, L., Hug C.C., Hatcher, C.R. Anesthesiology 59:132-138, 1983.
27. Ramsay J.G., Cutfield, G.R., Francis, C.M., Devlin, W.H., Foex, P. Br. J. Anaesth. 58:321-326, 1986.
28. Priebe, H.J., Skarvan, K.: Anesthesiology 66:114-121, 1987.
29. Videcoq, M., Arvieux, C.C., Ramsay, J.G., Foex, P., et al.: Anesthesiology, in press, 1987.
30. Tosone, S.R., Reves, J.G., Kissin, I., Smith, L.R., Fornier, S.E. Anesth. Analg. 62:903-908, 1983.
31. Kates, R.A., Zaggy, A.P., Norfleet, E.A., Health, K.R. Anesthesiology 61:10-18, 1984.
32. Pedersen, J.L., Strom, J., Berthelsen, P., Eriksen, J., Rasmussen, J.P. Acta Anaesthesiol. Scand. 29:354-357, 1985.
33. Chew, C.Y.C., Hect, S., McAllister, R.G., Singh, B.H. Am. J. Cardiol. 47:917-922, 1981.
34. Vatner, S.F., Higgins, C.B., Ratouck, P., Franklin, D., Braunwald, E. J. Clin. Invest. 50:2585-2595, 1971.
35. Vatner, S.F. Environ. Health Perspect. 26:193-206, 1978.
36. Bonow, R.O., Rosing, D.R., Epstein, S.E. Eur. Heart J. 4(Suppl F):57-65, 1983.
37. Henling, C.E., Slogoff, S., Kodali, S.V., Arlund, C. Anesth. Analg. 63:515-520, 1984.
38. Chelly, J.E., Hysing, E.S., Abernethy, D., Doursout. M-F., Merin, R.G. Anesthesiology 65:266-271, 1986.
39. Chelly, J.E., Hysing, E.S., Abernethy, D.R., Doursout, M-F., Hartley, C.J., Guerret, Merin, R.G. J. Pharmacol. Exper. Ther. 241:899-906, 1987.
40. McAllister, Jr., R.G., Hamann, S.R., Blouin, R.A. Am. J. Cardiol. 55:30B-40B, 1985.
41. Gelman, S., Fowler, K.C., Smith, L.R. Anesthesiology 61:726-730, 1984.
42. Hughes, R.L., Campbell, D., Fitch, W. Br. J. Anaesth. 52:1079-1086, 1980.
43. Thomson, P.D., Melmon, K.L., Richardson, J.A., Coh, K., Steinbrunn, W., Cudihee, R., Rowland, M. Ann. Intern. Med. 78:499-508, 1973.

COMPLICATIONS ASSOCIATED WITH THE PLACEMENT OF THE PULMONARY ARTERY CATHETER

INTRODUCTION - THE PROBLEM

Since the early 1970's when Swan, Ganz and associates published their work on "bedside" right heart catheterization using a balloon flotation catheter, this technique has become widely used and accepted. The original publications on pulmonary artery (PA) catheterization led one to believe that this procedure was easy, safe, and effective.

While it may be true that once learned the PA catheter technique is usually easy to perform, it is now quite clear that there are potential life threatening risks involved. It is also quite clear that to date, no study has unequivocally documented improved outcome from use of the procedure in any patient population. This fact, however, is coupled with the fact that four out of every ten dying patients has PA catheterization performed as part of the "last rites" theraputic maneuvers.

Complications associated with the use of PA catheters occurs with a clinically significant frequency. Approximately one in every four patients in whom a PA catheter is used suffers some major problem from its use which subsequently requires theraputic intervention. Approximately 4% of the critically ill patients in whom a PA catheter is used dies as a result of a catheter induced complication.

PA catheter use is based upon a belief (faith) that it will provide physiological information that will guide and improve therapy and ultimately patient outcome. Robin has pointed out Silverman's explanation for the wide spread use of the PA catheter in critically ill patients. Together, these two authors point out the problem with such "faith".

> "The proponents of pulmonary flow catheters should be required to demonstrate their safety and effectiveness. Given

existing data, the most that could be hoped for is a barely favorable risk-benefit ratio in some subclasses of patients.

(There) is the feeling that almost any intervention is justified in the critically ill patient. Silverman...has proposed an interesting aphorism for those finding themselves in a fireworks factory: 'It is better to curse the darkness than to light the wrong candle.' It is clear that many of our critically ill patients find themselves 'in a fireworks factory.' It is probable that we frequently light the wrong candle."(9)

COMPLICATION ASSOCIATED WITH THE PLACEMENT OF THE PA CATHETER

Dysrhythmias

Dysrhythmias are the most common placement complication associated with use of the PA catheter. Dysrhythmias occur in as many as eight of every ten patients in whom the PA catheter is floated into position. Many varieties of dysrhythmia may occur including atrial and ventricular premature contractions, ventricular tachydysrhythmias and bundle branch blocks. Self limited ventricular tachycardia (VT) may occur in as many as one third of patients in whom a PA catheter is used. In 5% there may be sustained VT. Factors which increased the risk of the occurrence of VT include shock, acidosis, hypoxia, electrolyte imbalance, and prolonged time for PA catheterization.

Localized/Generalized Cardiovascular Damage

Localized damage to the heart, i.e., endocardial hemorrhage, endocarditis, thrombus formation, and generalized damage to the cardiovascular system, i.e., embolic phenomenon and sepsis, all occur as a result of the placement of the PA catheter, a foreign body, in the vascular tree. Endocardial hemorrhage and thrombus formation occurs more frequently (> 50% of patients) than is generally recognized. The incidence does not seem to be related to the length of time that the catheter is in place. Endocardial trauma and hemorrhage, more localized valve trauma and intracavitary thrombus formation all predispose patients to infective endocarditis and sepsis. When PA catheter tips are cultured there is a high incidence of bacterial growth. This is also unrelated to the length of time that the catheter is in place. While cardiac trauma and positive bacterial cultures are frequently seen, $<$ 10% of the patients develop infective endocarditis and/or sepsis. When considering potential sources of iatrogenic infection in PA catheter placement one must remember to focus upon; a) the transducer system for pressure measurement, b) the blood sampling protocol when PA catheters are used, for example, to measure mixed venous oxygen saturation, and c) the cardiac output measurement protocol during which injections into the PA catheter are performed.

Pulmonary Infarction

The incidence of pulmonary infarction secondary to PA catheter use approximates 7%. The causes of pulmonary infarction include a) pulmonary embolus secondary to thrombus formed along the catheter, b) direct pulmonary vascular occlusion by the catheter being wedged peripherally in the pulmonary circulation, and c) prolonged balloon inflation. Congestive heart failure, reduced cardiac output and reductions in pulmonary blood flow all contribute to the occurrence of pulmonary infarctions secondary to PA catheter placement. There is also an inherent tendency for the PA catheter to migrate to a peripheral location in the pulmonary circulation as a result of rhythmic cardiac contractions and the propelling force of pulsatile blood flow. This is especially true if a large loop of PA catheter exists in the right ventricle. It has been suggested that if balloon occlusion occurs with less than 1.5 ml of air, then the catheter tip is too far out and a loop may exist in the right ventricle, both of which indicate that the catheter could be pulled back until balloon occlusion occurs with a full 1.5 ml of air. It must also be remembered that when cardiac operations are performed, the surgeon's manipulation of the heart may cause the PA catheter to migrate distally requiring withdrawl of the catheter and proper positioning after surgery.

Pulmonary Artery Rupture

Pulmonary artery rupture is the most devastating of PA catheter complications. The incidence of this problem is 0.2%. Diagnosis of pulmonary artery rupture is made be identifying the following signs and symptoms: a) hemoptysis, b) $\downarrow$ BP, c) $\downarrow$ hematocrit, d) $\downarrow$ arterial oxygenation, e) dyspnea, f) bronchospasm, g) pleural effusion, h) hemothorax, i) pneumothorax, j) pulmonary infiltrate on chest x-ray, k) extravasation of contrast dye from the ruptured branch pulmonary artery when a pulmonary wedge angiogram is performed, 1) localized bleeding site identified at bronchoscopy. The differential diagnosis of pulmonary artery rupture secondary to PA catheter placement includes pulmonary edema pulmonary, infarction, and trauma to the tracheobronchial tree.

The pathogenesis of pulmonary artery rupture is understood by considering the components of the PA catheter tip. The tip of the catheter itself may puncture the artery as can excessive pressure in the balloon. If the balloon inflates in eccentric fashion it may expose the catheter tip and predispose it to puncture the vessel. The risk of arterial rupture increases in patients > 60 years of age. It is unclear whether pulmonary artery hypertension increases the risk of arterial rupture although there is some evidence that supports this notion.

Prevention of pulmonary artery rupture secondary to PA catheter placement requires meticulous attention to catheter tip placement avoiding peripheral location and balloon overinflation. Special precautions must be considered during cardiac surgery when the PA catheter becomes stiff with induced hypothermia. If the balloon remains inflated for a prolonged time, the problems with expanding gas volume must be considered and dealt with if nitrous oxide is being administered.

Treatment of pulmonary artery rupture secondary to PA catheter placement is difficult at best. The offending catheter can be withdrawn and the patient positioned with the affected lung down to protect the unaffected lung from blood aspiration. Supportive therapy includes a) administration of oxygen, b) measures to minimize coughing and straining, c) avoidence of airway suctioning if possible and, d) drugs to ↓ PA pressure. PEEP may tamponade the bleeding. More drastic hemorrhage may necessitate the placement of a double lumen tube to separate and isolate the lungs and/or surgical hemostasis.

SUMMARY

"In the last analysis, the widespread use of pulmonary flow catheters, like many other practices in medicine, is a form of cultism. Based on a series of unsupported beliefs the practice has become widely adopted. Growth has been fostered by an uncritical literature and widely spread by means of oral communication. Only recently has an estimate of the nature and amount of harm associated with the catheter become possible. It is clean that risks are high. The potential benefits for most patients are much less than is currently appreciated. Individual physicians should do their own risk-benefit analysis before exposing their patients to the use of pulmonary artery flow catheters"[9].

Suggested Readings

1. Abernathy WS: Chest:349, 1974
2. Barash PG, Nardi D, Hammond G, et al.: J Thorac Cardiovasc Surg 82:5-12, 1981
3. Elliott CG, Zimmerman GA, Clemmer TP: Chest 76:647-652, 1979
4. Foote GA, Schabel SI, Hodges M: N Engl J Med 290:927-931, 1974
5. McDaniel DD, Stone JG, Faltas AN, et al.: J Thorac Cardiovasc Surg 82:1-4, 1981
6. Muller BJ, Gallucci A: Can Anaesth Joc J 32:258-264, 1985
7. Pape LA, Haffajee CI, Markis JE, et al.: Ann Int Med 90:344-347, 1979
8. Patel C, Laboy V, Venus B, et al.: Crit Care Med 14:195-197, 1986
9. Robin ED: Ann Int Med 103:445-449, 1985
10. Rowley KM, Sini Clubb K, Smith GJW, et al.: N Engl J Med 311:1152-1156, 1984
11. Sprung CL, Jacobs LJ, Caralis PV, et al.: Chest 79:413-415, 1981
12. Swan HJC, Ganz W, Forrester J, et al.: N Engl J Med 283:447-451, 1970

NON-INVASIVE MONITORING

P. BARASH

I. INTRODUCTION

Invasive cardiovascular monitoring facilitates the diagnosis and treatment of complex hemodynamic disorders. These can be categorized in terms of: pump function, intravascular volume, and vascular resistance. Although the benefit of these techniques is important for patient care, limitations are now becoming obvious. The risk associated with invasive monitoring poses a potentially significant hazard to the critically ill patient. Further, most invasive cardiac monitoring is based upon the assumption that pressure measurements are a good approximation of ventricular volume status (preload). Erroneous conclusions based on this notion of hemodynamic performance may result. Consequently, non-invasive techniques will be used with greater frequency to improve diagnostic capability while reducing risk to the patient.[1]

II. ELECTROCARDIOGRAM (ECG)

Although the ECG is a direct measure of the heart's electrical activity, it also indirectly yields important information regarding cardiac pump function. For example, a nodal rhythm with the concommitant loss of atrial contraction can result in significant decreases (10-15%) in cardiac output. The electrocardiogram (ECG) supplies an enormous amount of information regarding the status of the coronary circulation. By use of a calibrated ECG (10 mm = 1 mV) employing leads V5/II, 96% of EKG detectable ischemic events can be diagnosed. ECG changes seen with ischemia include both ST segment changes and arrhythmias. However, electrocardiographic changes are usually a late sign of ischemia. Changes in ventricular compliance and regional wall motion precede ST changes.[2] Newer directions in intraoperative ECG monitoring will be aided by computer assisted analysis of ischemia (ST segments) and arrhythmias. Kotrly et al. have demonstrated the utility of an ST segment trending system which facilitates earlier recognition of myocardial ischemia.[3]

This assumes even greater importance, when the anesthesiologist is confronted with a patient who has "silent" myocardial ischemia. A notion exists that an "awake" patient, under a regional anesthetic (spinal or peridural), is a sensitive indicator of myocardial ischemia. Recent evidence suggests that this concept is incorrect and may lead to significant morbidity. A number of studies have documented the incidence of "silent ischemia" or asymptomatic coronary artery disease.[4] This entity can be defined as: the absence of angina (or its equivalents) in the presence of objective evidence of transient myocardial ischemia (EKG, radionuclear or echocardiographic studies, etc.). Three groups of patients may present with this disease process:

(a) Totally asymptomatic patients
(b) Asymptomatic patients post-myocardial infarction (MI) who have active ischemia
(c) Patients with angina who are asymptomatic with some ischemic episodes, but not with others.

At present, approximately two to four percent of asymptomatic males (greater than 45 years of age) and 20-30% of asymptomatic post MI patients have episodes of silent ischemia. The incidence of "silent" S-T segment depression (EKG) is quite high. More than 2/3 of ischemic events are undetected by "awake" patients. To further complicate matters, many of these events are not accompanied by significant alterations in heart rate or blood pressure. Slogoff and Keats have reported similar findings in a group of anesthetized patients undergoing coronary artery bypass surgery.[5] Only one third of these ischemic events were associated with hemodynamic abnormalities. A number of awake patients with silent ischemia have a "defective anginal warning system". It appears they have an altered perception of pain. On a theoretical basis, treatment with sedative or analgesic medications may further decrease their ability to perceive angina.

III. INDIRECT BLOOD PRESSURE

Non-invasive measurement of blood pressure (BP) is basic to the practice of anesthesia. At present, four major techniques are available for indirect measurement:

1. Oscillation
2. Auscultation (Korotkoff sounds)
3. Ultrasonic detection arterial wall movement (Doppler)
4. Blood flow detection distal to cuff (palpation, Doppler, photoelectric)

Despite numerous studies reporting a high correlation between non-invasive and intra-arterial monitoring, arterial catheterization continues to be widely practiced for the higher risk patient where (1) beat-to-beat measurement of blood pressure is important and (2) sampling of arterial blood (for blood gases, chemistries, etc.) is essential. However, even with invasive arterial monitoring, the clinician may receive inaccurate information. In addition, the risk of clinically significant complications are always present. To offset these limitations, the clinician will have non-invasive devices that measure BP on a beat-to-beat basis. Applicable to anesthesia practice is the use of a finger mounted BP cuff ("Penaz method") which allows beat-to-beat BP determination under a wide variety of clinical circumstances.[6]

If non-invasive BP measurement is to achieve popularity, a method must be available to non-invasively monitor "ABG's". Commercially available transcutaneous monitoring accurately measures of pO_2 and pCO_2 in both neonates <u>and</u> adults. Alternatively, pulse oximetry combined with measurements of end tidal CO_2 may offer the clinician a "substitute" for ABGs. (See sections by K. Tremper, M.D., Ph.D.).

IV. <u>CARDIAC PERFORMANCE</u>

A. <u>Nuclear Cardiology</u>

Evaluation of dynamic cardiac function can be performed with radioactive tracers (radionuclides) that remain in the intravascular space during the period of study. An excellent review of this topic has recently appeared in <u>Anesthesiology</u> by Cahalan et al.[7]

Radionuclear evaluation has also highlighted some of the potential hemodynamic pitfalls inherent in postoperative care. To evaluate preload, PCWP is commonly used as an indirect measurement of left ventricular end diastolic pressure (LVEDP). Based upon this information ventricular function curves are constructed, which assume that LVEDP (or PCWP) and left ventricular end diastolic volume (LVEDV) have a direct linear relationship. However, investigations have shown that under a wide variety of circumstances commonly encountered in the ICU, PCWP, and LVEDV do not correlate.[8-9]

B. Echocardiography

Echocardiography requires the use of a transducer, which is both the transmitter and receiver.[1,7,10] The typical transducer, a piezoelectric crystal, transmits a beam of sound which may be reflected, refracted or transmitted when it encounters an interface between acoustic media of different densities. The transducer emits sound of high frequency, 1-10 million cycles/second (Hz), for 1 microsecond and receives for the remaining 999 microseconds. Since the speed of sound (1540 m/sec) is fairly constant for heart and surrounding tissues, the distance between the reflecting surface and the transducer can be derived from the elapsed time between propagation and reception of the signal by the transducer.

M mode echocardiography (motion mode) uses a thin beam of sound to create an "ice pick" view of the heart. In another words, it generates a "one dimensional recording" that lacks spatial orientation. Although, the M mode is referred to as a "one dimension" technique, the second dimension, time, is extremely important for interpretation.

To overcome the inherent spatial difficulties, two dimensional or cross sectional echocardiographic techniques have been developed. Two dimensional echocardiography (2DE) uses multiple beams of sound in the form of a pie shaped section to construct larger, spatially correct images of the heart. This is important in patients with coronary artery disease, since M mode echocardiography may "miss" dyskinetic areas due to the narrow area the sound beam penetrates.

Global left ventricular performance is evaluated by measurement of end diastolic and end systolic dimensions. From these dimensions, estimates of ventricular volume, cardiac output, ejection fraction, mean circumferential fiber shortening rate, and systolic time intervals can be obtained. Excellent correlation between echocardiographic data and results of angiographic determinations of these variable in adults and children has been reported. However, at present, caution must still be exercised in the use of echocardiography for estimation of ventricular size and performance. It is implicit in these techniques that certain geometric and physiologic assumptions are made converting a two-dimensional echocardiographic measurement to an estimate of left ventricular volume. The strengths of echocardiography lie in the ability to make combined anatomic and physiologic diagnoses.

Although radionuclear studies expose the patient to radiation, ultrasound carries no known risk. This lack of risk has enabled detailed examination of the physiologic changes in cardiovascular function of the parturient.[1] Information obtained from these examinations will allow the anesthesiologist, obstetrician and pediatrician to formulate plans for management of pregnancy, delivery and the postnatal period.

Studies in the OR using echocardiography, were originally performed with M mode echocardiography. By use of M mode echocardiography, we found a 28% decrease in cardiac output in children anesthetized with halothane (2%) and N_2O/O_2. Administration of atropine resulted in prompt increase in cardiac output by 47%.[11]

Newer studies have highlighted the use of transesophageal echocardiography (TEE) in a group of patients with coronary artery disease. Early detection of ischemia may be facilitated by TEE, since development of regional wall abnormalities are an immediate consequence of ischemia. In a study comparing electrocardiography and 2D TEE, Smith et al. concluded that echocardiography was a superior method for detecting intraoperative myocardial ischemia.[12] Further, when new segmental wall motion abnormalities persist, a myocardial infarction is likely to have occurred. Clements and deBrujin have recently received this topic in detail.[13]

Postoperatively, echocardiography can not only aid in the diagnosis of "ventricular interference", but also help in the selection of the optimum level of PEEP.[14-15] Usually, an increase in PCWP and decrease in cardiac output (CO) can be interpreted as LV failure. However, under certain circumstances, an elevated PCWP and decreased CO may be a grossly misleading indicator of LV performance. As the interventricular septum encroaches on the LV cavity these hemodynamic data may actually reflect decreased filling volume of the left ventricle! Rather than limiting fluid administration, which would be the management in congestive heart failure, treatment is directed at reducing PAP and normalizing right ventricular volume. Jardin and colleagues, in an elegant study using 2-D echocardiography, followed the leftward shift of the interventricular septum (IVS) in response to increasing levels of PEEP (0-30 cmH_2O). They reported the decrease in cardiac output is mediated by a displacement of the IVS rather than decreased venous return. The authors concluded that at higher levels of PEEP, volume loading has a limited role. Further, inotropic support is of questionable value since left ventricular function is normal, but diastolic compliance is altered.

Two new enhancements to 2D echocardiography will increase the value of this monitor to clinicians in the perioperative period. Doppler echocardiography utilizing either pulsed wave (single ultrasound crystal acts as a transmitter and receiver) or continuous wave (2 separate crystals) allows quantification of the direction and velocity of blood flow in cardiac chambers or the aorta. Thus, intraoperative assessment of: valve function (stenosis or regurgitation), cardiac output, intracardiac shunts and indirect measurement of intracardiac pressures can be obtained.[16] Further, the addition of color flow mapping enhances the utility of the Doppler examination. Previously, Doppler echocardiography allowed real time measurement of flow at single point in the cardiac chamber. Color flow technology allows measurement of the whole aspect of intrachamber blood flow. Color-encoded, digitalized multigated signals are analyzed by computer in real time. Flow toward the transducer is red, while flow directed away from the transducer is blue. Relative velocities are depicted by eight shades of color; the higher the velocity, the lighter the shade. Green represents turbulent flow.[17]

V. CONCLUSIONS

Rather than being the monitoring of the future, non-invasive devices offer clinician an immense amount of data which can positively influence patient care during preoperative evaluation, in the operating room and the intensive care unit. Even as this subject is being presented, newer non-invasive methods such as nuclear magnetic resonance (NMR) are being developed.[18] Just as invasive monitoring, (e.g. Swan-Ganz catheter) has raised our "awareness" of cardiovascular physiology, these non-invasive methods offer a unique method of supplementing our knowledge of the cardiovascular system.

However, the best non-invasive monitor is OBSERVATION by the clinician, who uses monitoring to supplement and aid clinical decision making, rather than have the "numbers" dictate clinical practice!!!

BIBLIOGRAPHY

1. Reitan J, Barash P: Non-invasive Monitoring. In: Monitoring in Anesthesia. L Saidman, NT Smith, Second Edition, 1984, Butterworth: England, pp 117-191.

2. Barash PG: Monitoring myocardial oxygen balance: Physiologic basis and clinical application. Refresher Courses in Anesthesiology 13:21-32, 1985.
3. Kotrly K, Kotter GS, Mortara D, et al.: Intraoperative detection of myocardial ischemia with ST segment trend monitoring system. Anesth Analg 63:343-345, 1984.
4. Cohn PF: Silent myocardial ischemia: Present status. Mod Conc Cardiovasc Dis 56:1-5, 1987.
5. Slogoff S, Keats AS: Further observations on perioperative myocardial ischemia. Anesthesiology 5:539-542, 1986.
6. Smith NT, Wesseling KH, de Wit B: Evaluation of two prototype devices producing non-invasive, pulsatile, calibrated blood pressure measurement from a finger. J Clin Monitoring 1:17-29, 1985.
7. Cahalan MK, Litt L, Botvinick EH, Schiller NB: Advances in non-invasive cardiovascular imaging: Implications for the anesthesiologist. Anesthesiology 66:356-372, 1987.
8. Calvin JE, Driedger AA, Sibbald WJ: Does the pulmonary capillary wedge pressure predict left ventricular preload in critically ill patients? Crit Care Med 9:437-443, 1981.
9. Hansen RM, Viquerat CE, Matthay MA, et al. Poor correlation between pulmonary arterial wedge pressure and left ventricular end diastolic volume after coronary artery bypass graft surgery. Anesthesiology 64:764-770, 1986.
10. LaMantia KR, Lehmann KG, Barash PG: Echocardiography in the Perioperative period. Acute Care 11:106-116, 1985.
11. Barash PG, Glanz S, Katz JD, et al.: Ventricular function in children during halothane anesthesia: an echocardiographic evaluation. Anesthesiology 49:79-85, 1978.
12. Smith JS, Cahalan MK, Benefiel DJ, et al.: Intraoperative detection of myocardial ischemia in high risk patients: electrocardiography versus two dimensional transesophageal echocardiography. Circulation 72:1015-1021, 1985.
13. Clements FM, de Bruijn NP: Perioperative evaluation of regional wall motion by transesophageal two dimensional echocardiography. Anesth Analg 66:249-261, 1987.

14. Jardin F, Farcot JC, Boisante L, et al.: Influence of positive end expiratory pressure on left ventricular performance. 304:387-392, 1981.
15. Laver MB, Strauss HW, Pohost GM: Right and left ventricular geometry: Adjustments during acute respiratory failure. Crit Care Med 7:509-519, 1979.
16. Nishimura RA, Miller FA, Callahan MJ: Doppler echocardiography: Theory, instrumentation, technique and application. Mayo Clin Proc 60:321-343, 1985.
17. Myatake K, Okamoto M, Kinoshita N, et al.: Clinical applications of a new type of real-time two-dimensional doppler flow imaging system. Am J Cardiol 54:857-868, 1984.
18. Kaufman L, Crooks L, Sheldon P, et al.: The potential impact of nuclear magnetic resonance imaging on cardiovascular diagnosis. Circulation 67:251-257, 1983.

HISTAMINE RELEASE AND NEUROMUSCULAR BLOCKING DRUGS: CLINICAL PHARMACOLOGY AND CIRCULATORY MECHANISMS

J. J. SAVARESE, M.D.

BACKGROUND

Histamine release by neuromuscular blocking drugs may occur by two mechanisms: (1) a true hypersensitivity reaction involving immune mechanisms; (2) a pharmacological response which is dose-related and which is due to a type of displacement of mast cell contents. The latter mechanism will be discussed during this lecture.

Pharmacological histamine release is still surprisingly poorly understood by anesthesiologists. The clinical pharmacology of minor to moderate degrees of histamine release has only recently been quantified in the case of both neuromuscular blocking drugs and narcotic analgesics. The results of these measurements should place the response in proper clinical perspective. In certain cases, the response may be used to advantage as a method of circulatory manipulation.

PHARMACOLOGY OF HISTAMINE

H_1 receptors mediate H_1 blockers prevent	bronchospasm, gut contraction, vascular dilatation, capillary permeability
H_2 receptors mediate H_2 blockers prevent	gastric acid secretion, myocardial inotropism and chronotropism, vascular dilatation, bronchodilation

METABOLISM OF HISTAMINE

This subject is pertinent to a discussion of histamine release, since a number of maneuvers, by slowing metabolism and elimination of histamine, may accentuate the histamine release response.

There are two major metabolic pathways:

(1) Ring methylation (via histamine N-methyltransferase) - major pathway in man

(2) Oxidative deamination (via diamine oxidase)

Metabolites are excreted in the urine.

These drugs especially may accentuate a histamine-release response:

(1) Cimetidine (less so ranitidine) - inhibits histamine N-methyltransferase. H_2 blockers also prevent a negative feedback mechanism which operates normally to minimize histamine liberation.

(2) Droperidol - inhibits N-methyltransferase

(3) Beta-blockers - inhibit circulatory compensatory mechanisms.

HISTAMINE RELEASE BY NEUROMUSCULAR BLOCKING DRUGS

Although recognized for a long time, the response was first quantified by Moss et al for d-tubocurarine (ref. 1). In this study, histamine release was found to be dose-related, a pharmacological response. The degree of fall in blood pressure was directly related to rise in serum histamine. Curare's hypotensive property can be entirely attributed to histamine release.

Subsequent studies with a variety of drugs (ref. 6, 9, 10) have shown that the response is very sensitive to speed of injection, and that combinations of H_1 and H_2 blockers will shift the dose-response curve to the right in man by a factor of about two.

Studies correlating clinical cardiovascular response with serum histamine level have often used maximal fall in blood pressure as the clinical indicator. In my opinion, this correlation, although useful, dramatically overestimates the clinical significance of the response because the fall in blood pressure is so short-lived. For example, a 40 percent fall in arterial pressure may sound rather ominous until the qualification is made that the interval during which arterial pressure is less than 80 percent of control is less than one-half minute! Various aspects of this topic will be discussed in detail in order to place the response in proper perspective.

TAKING ADVANTAGE OF THE HISTAMINE RELEASE RESPONSE

A brief (1-3) minute period of vasodilatation develops during a moderate histamine release response. This is accompanied by increased myocardial inotropy and chronotropy (via H_2 receptors). Peripheral vasodilatation results in increased cardiac output with little or no increase in myocardial work. Thus, the modest effect of a longer-acting drug like d-tubocurarine may be additive with other peripheral vasodilators when induced hypotension is contemplated.

The brief fall in arterial pressure may also be useful to counteract excessive reactive hypertension during intubation of the trachea in particularly susceptible individuals such as patients with hypertensive cardiovascular disease.

REFERENCES

1. Moss, J., Rosow, C.E., Savarese, J.J., Philbin, D.M., Kniffen, K.J. Anesthesiology 55:19-25, 1981.
2. Lorenz, W., Doenicke, A. Mt. Sinai Med J (NY) 45:357-386, 1978.
3. Beavan, M.A. Monogr Allergy 13:1-114, 1978.
4. Savarese, J.J. Anesthesiology 50:40-46, 1979.
5. Moss, J., Philbin, D.M, Rosow, C.E., Basta, S.J. et al. Klin Wochenschr 60:891-895, 1982.
6. Philbin, D.M., Moss, J., Akins, C.W., Rosow, C.E. et al. Anesthesiology 55:292-296, 1981.
7. Savarese, J.J., Ali, H.H., Basta, S.J., Sunder, N. et al. Anesthesiology 58:333-341, 1983.
8. Basta, S.J., Savarese, J.J., Ali, H.H. et al. Anesth Analg (Cleve) 61:723-724, 1982.
9. Scott, R.P.F., Savarese, J.J., Basta, S.J., Embree, P.B. et al. Br J Anaesth 58:834-838, 1986.
10. Basta, B.J., Savarese, J.J., Ali, H.H., Moss J. et al. Br J Anaesth 55:105S, 1983.
11. Scott, R.P.F., Savarese, J.J., Ali, H.H., Gargarian, M. et al. Br J Anaesth 54:909-913, 1985.

ANESTHESIA AND THE AGING HEART

R. MERIN

If "aged" is defined as greater than 65 years old, then at the present time approximately 11% of the United States population, or 25 million persons, fall into this category. It may be likely that within their lifetime 50% of these individuals will need anesthesia and surgery. Consequently, it is understandable that there has been a good deal of attention paid recently to the problem of anesthesia in the geriatric population. Although there is somewhat more published data on other aspects of anesthesia and the older patient, as will become evident, there is great sparsity of solid data looking at the effect of anesthesia and anesthetics on cardiovascular function in the aged, and particularly comparing this effect with a younger population. Perhaps the cardiovascular effects of aging are not that important. In fact, it has been suggested that the major diseases interfering with physical activity in the aged population are non-cardiac (1). What then are the cardiovascular effects of aging?

EFFECTS OF AGE ON THE CARDIOVASCULAR SYSTEM

Although it has been said that cardiac output is 35% less at the age of 70 than at 20 years (2) or that maximum cardiac output decreases at a rate of 1% per year from the middle of the fifth decade of life onwards with heart rate decreasing by about half that rate (2), in fact, it would appear that these observations may be a function of disease and environment (3). Non-invasive longitudinal studies have shown that as the healthy individual ages, there is no change in resting heart rate nor in the response to rather substantial work loads. However, the mechanism of maintaining heart rate does vary between the young and old. Whereas the young tend to increase their cardiac output in response to stress by increasing their heart rate with little change in stroke volume or end-diastolic volume, the elderly predominantly increase cardiac output under these circumstances by increasing their ventricular filling pressures and volumes (13). The mechanism behind these changes is probably two-fold. In the first place, as we age, there are definite anatomic changes in our resistance arteries with increased water and fibrous tissue content and less elasticity leading to progressively increasing systemic vascular resistance. In order to maintain cardiac output, the aged cardiovascular system responds with increasing preload. One of the reasons for this is that there is reasonable evidence in both animals and man that although the activity of the sympathetic nervous system does not change appreciably with age, and in fact may even increase (plasma catecholamines), the response to this sympathetic stimulation definitely does decrease so that even with increasing sympathetic nervous system activation, there is little response of heart rate and cardiac contractility. Of further interest in both aging animals and humans, the observed deterioration in large patient populations in cardiovascular function can be prevented or even reversed by conditioning and exercise programs (3). Of course, as we age there is an increased incidence of cardiovascular diseases (4). Consequently, the effects of aging on the cardiovascular system must encompass not only chronologic age but also the effects of environment and disease.

EFFECTS OF ANESTHETICS ON THE HEALTHY CARDIOVASCULAR SYSTEM

Inhalation Anesthetics. The currently available potent inhalation anesthetics, halothane, enflurane, and isoflurane, have similar effects on the cardiovascular system in healthy humans. In general, with increasing dose, all three anesthetics produce a decrease in cardiac output, stroke volume and systemic vascular resistance. However, there appear to be quantitative differences. Halothane has minimal effects on heart rate whereas both enflurane and isoflurane tend to produce increases in heart rate although not dose related. Although high concentrations of halothane and enflurane can produce a decrease in systemic vascular resistance, clinical concentrations usually have little effect on the peripheral vascular system. On the other hand, there is a dose-related decrease in systemic vascular resistance produced by isoflurane. Partly as a result of this, equi-potent anesthetic concentrations of isoflurane produce less decrease in cardiac output than those seen with halothane and enflurane. In both animals and man, all three potent inhalation anesthetics cause marked interference in the normal baroreflex control of the cardiovascular system (4).

Intravenous Drugs Used in Anesthesia. Intravenous drugs used in anesthesia have not been as rigorously studied for their effect on the cardiovascular system. However, in general, the hypnotic drugs, especially the barbiturates, tend to produce predominantly systemic vasodilation often accompanied by reflex tachycardia, although if given in large doses rapidly, direct depression of cardiac output can also occur. The major exception to this generalization is etomidate. The predominant advantage of this drug is its lack of cardiovascular depressant qualities. The anesthetic benzodiazopines, of which there are a variety available in Europe, but only diazepam and midazolam in this country, also produce predominantly vasodilation with minimal effects on cardiac output. Likewise, anesthetic doses of the opiate receptor agonists, especially morphine and the fentanyl derivatives, produce varying degrees of vasodilation with minimal effects on cardiac function. The unique intravenous anesthetic drug, ketamine, is also unique as far as its cardiovascular effects are concerned. Ketamine routinely produces cardiovascular stimulation with increases in heart rate, systemic pressures and cardiac output.

Regional Anesthesia. As long as direct systemic administration of large (toxic) doses of local anesthetics are avoided, the cardiovascular effects of regional anesthesia are minimal. Even spinal or epidural anesthesia as high as T1-3 produces predominantly a decrease in systemic vascular resistance (5). However, there does appear to be some interference in normal baroreflex responses even in young individuals (6).

CARDIOVASCULAR EFFECTS OF ANESTHESIA IN THE AGED

Animal Studies. To my knowledge, the only animal investigation comparing the effects of an anesthetic in a young and aged population studied the effects of halothane in young and aged rats (7). As had been demonstrated in humans, the anesthetic requirement for halothane was almost 20% lower in the aged than in the young rats. When the animals were studied at equi-anesthetic doses, arterial blood pressure and heart rate, both awake and at all anesthetic concentrations, were lower in the aged rats. Regional blood flow was also generally different in the aged rats. For instance, renal blood flow was lower awake but was not affected by anesthesia in either group. Myocardial blood flow was also significantly lower awake and at all anesthetic concentrations except for the highest at which point aged and young rats' myocardial blood flow was the same. Cerebral blood flow did not differ in the two populations awake but the increase seen within increasing concentrations of halothane in the young animals was not seen in the aged animals. Of considerable interest is the fact that 4 of the 10 aged rats died during the high concentrations of halothane while none of the 13 young rats succumbed (even though the high concentration of halothane was 20% greater in the young rats). Thus, even accounting for the increased CNS potency of halothane in the aged rat, the cardiovascular effects particularly with high concentrations were markedly accentuated, even to the point of death.

Human Studies. For, I suppose, obvious reasons, there have been no studies of the effect of anesthetics on healthy aged volunteers as we have available for the young population. In fact, there is a paucity of studies in which the same group of investigators compared the effects of the same anesthetics in a young and aged population. I am aware of only four. Haldemann and co-workers studied the effects of a clinical anesthetic sequence using enflurane as the predominant anesthetic (8). They compared a group of 15 young, healthy patients aged 20-40 years with 7 elderly patients aged 60-80 years. A lower concentration of enflurane was used in the elderly (1-1.6%) than in the young (1.6-2%). 66% nitrous oxide was also used. During anesthesia, there was significantly more decrease in cardiac output and arterial pressure in the aged patients. With surgical stimulation, arterial pressure increased in the aged population so that it was equal to the younger population, but cardiac output and heart rate remained depressed. The other studies in which the same investigators compared young and aged populations were performed by Christensen et al (9-11). They compared the effects of an induction dose of thiopental in a young and elderly patient population. They also separated their patient population by sex. In both male and female, the induction dose for loss of consciousness was lower in the elderly group. Likewise in both populations there was minimal difference of the effect of thiopental on cardiovascular performance in the young and old. However, in both young and aged women, thiopental produced a significant decrease in cardiac output whereas in neither young and aged men was there a change in cardiac output produced by thiopental. Finally, Bergenwald and colleagues studied the effects of spinal anesthesia with tetracaine in both a young (5) and an aged (12) population. However, note that these studies were separated by almost 10 years. In addition, in the young group, a larger dose of tetracaine produced a considerably higher block, T1-3 versus T8-10 in the aged population. They also looked at the effect of a vasoconstrictor, dihydroergotamine, but only used half the dose in the elderly population. In addition, some of their patients in the aged group were in their 40's! Given these differences in the experimental design, the following results were reported. There was more decrease in cardiac output, stroke volume and mean arterial pressure in the aged population than in the younger population even though the level of the block was considerably lower. In both groups, both right and left ventricular filling pressures were significantly decreased by the spinal anesthetic. The response to dihydroergotamine, however, was very similar. The drug produced mostly peripheral arterial and veno-constriction with resulting correction in the hypotension but only partial correction of decrease in cardiac output in the elderly group and, in fact, a further decrease in cardiac output in the young group. In the elderly group the response to a 10-15° head-up tilt was also tested before and after the spinal anesthesia and after the vasoconstrictor. Awake tilt produced no change in heart rate or arterial pressure but decreases in cardiac output and stroke volume. After spinal anesthesia, marked decreases in mean arterial pressure and cardiac output occurred. All these changes were reversed by dihydroergotamine. Although Samii's group only measured arterial pressure and heart rate responses to low thoracic epidural anesthesia, they did note that whereas a T4-10 block produced no significant decrease in mean arterial pressure in a young group of patients (6), a T8-10 block produced more than a 30% decrease in mean arterial pressure in a group of elderly patients (13) confirming Bergenwald's observations that the elderly population responds to major conduction anesthesia with more cardiovascular depression.

Another reasonable design approach to compare effects of anesthetics in the elderly population would be for the same group of investigators to look at different anesthetics. Haldemann and co-workers, using the same experimental design as in comparing young and old patients anesthetized with nitrous oxide-enflurane (see above), also studied nitrous oxide-halothane and a neurolept anesthesia technique. The effects of halothane-nitrous oxide and neurolept anesthesia were similar with moderate decreases in cardiac output after induction of anesthesia which was maintained after surgical incision. Stroke volume was better maintained with neurolept anesthesia, although heart rate decreased. Cardiac output and stroke volume were less after anesthesia and after surgery with enflurane than with the other two anesthetics, whereas there was little difference between depression in mean arterial pressure and recovery of mean arterial pressure upon surgical incision.

The only other group to specifically study the effect of aging was Stefansson and co-workers from Sweden (15-17) who reported on the cardiovascular effects of several different anesthetic agents and techniques in elderly patients requiring surgery for hip fracture. They only reported two sets of data points, one after premedication with a small dose of droperidal and the other as the surgery was being completed. They compared ketamine, halothane, enflurane, a neurolept analgesic technique, and epidural anesthesia. Neurolept analgesia and epidural resulted in no significant change in any cardiovascular parameter (heart rate, arterial pressure, left ventricular filling pressure, cardiac index, stroke volume index, systemic vascular resistance, and pulmonary vascular resistance). Ketamine produced in increases in arterial pressure and cardiac index with no significant change in the other measured variables while both halothane and enflurane depressed arterial pressure with equivalent decreases in cardiac index and stroke volume. There were no perioperative deaths and minimal morbidity. The series of studies by Reiz and co-workers from Umea, Sweden, although directed at patients with ischemic heart disease, predominantly involved elderly patients (18-23). Their studies were after induction of anesthesia before surgical stimulation. In addition, the patients tended to have other cardiovascular diseases including hypertension and congestive heart failure. Consequently, they were considerably sicker than the other aged patients referred to thus far. Under these circumstances, induction of anesthesia with halothane (21), enflurane (23), isoflurane (22), thiopental (19), and thoracic epidural anesthesia (18) resulted in major decreases in mean arterial pressure (30% with thiopental and 40-50% with the other anesthetics). Although all three inhalation anesthetics produced significant (30-40%) decreases in vascular resistance as well, there was also a significant decrease in cardiac index and interestingly enough, in left ventricular filling pressure. Enflurane and isoflurane were administered in subanesthetic concentrations while halothane was given in anesthetic concentrations. Thiopental and neurolept analgesia (20) both maintained cardiac output at awake levels even though stroke volume was decreased because of increases in heart rate. The effect of thoracic epidural was remarkably similar to the potent inhalation anesthetics with a significant decrease in cardiac and stroke volume index as well as the hypotension (18).

Although there are a number of other isolated studies looking at the effects of anesthetics on cardiovascular function, it is difficult to draw conclusions from these studies and in addition, a number of them suffered from flawed techniques. From the limited information available on the effect of anesthetics on the aging heart, I would conclude, (1) in almost every instance, the dose of the anesthetic necessary for the same effect in the aged population was less than in the younger population; (2) the potent inhalation anesthetics appear to be more depressant to the cardiovascular system at lower concentrations in the aged population; (3) the intravenous drugs studied appear to show little difference in their effects on the cardiovascular system in young and aged populations; (4) epidural and spinal anesthesia appear to have more prominent cardiovascular effects in the aged population than in the younger population.

REFERENCES

1. Geer, R.T. Seminars in Anesthesia 5:23-30, 1986.

2. Hilgenberg, J.C. Seminars in Anesthesia 5:44-53, 1986.
3. Lakatta, E.G., Fleg, J.L. In Geriatric Anesthesia, Principles and Practice, ed. C.R. Stephen, R.A.E. Assaf, Butterworths, Boston, 1986, pp. 1-26.
4. Merin, R.G. In Geriatric Anesthesia, Principles and Practice, ed. C.R. Stephen, R.A.E. Assaf, Butterworths, Boston, 1986, pp. 219-242.
5. Bergenwald, L., Eklund, B., Kaijser, L., Klingenstrom, P., Westermark, L. Acta Anaesthesiol. Scand. 16:235-239, 1972.
6. Baron, J-F., Decaux-Jacolot, A., Edouard, A., et al. Anesthesiology 64:188-193, 1986.
7. Hoffman, W.E., Miletich, D.J., Albrecht, R.E., et al. Anesthesiology 56:444-448, 1982.
8. Haldemann, G., Schmid, E., Frey, P., et al. Anaesthesist 24:343-6, 1975.
9. Christensen, J.H., Andreasen, F., Jansen, J.A. Br. J. Anaesth. 55:33-30, 1983.
10. Ibid. Anaesthesia 37:398-404, 1982.
11. Christensen, J.H., Andreasen, F., Kristofforsen, M.B. Br. J. Anaesth. 55:391-7, 1983.
12. Bergenwald, L., Freyschuss, U., Kaijser, L., Westermark, L. Clin. Physiol. 1:453-460, 1981.
13. Ecoffey, C., Edouard, A., Pruszcynski, W., et al. Anesthesiology 62:294-7, 1985.
14. Haldemann, G., Hossli, G., Schaer, H. Anaesthesist 26:168-71, 1977.
15. Stefansson, T., Wickstrom, I., Haljamae, H. Acta Anaesthesiol. Scand. 26:371-7, 1982.
16. Ibid. Acta Anaesthesiol. Scand. 26:386-92, 1982.
17. Ibid. Acta Anaesthesiol. Scand. 26:378-85, 1982.
18. Reiz, S., Nath, S., Rais, O. Acta Anaesth. Scand. 24:11-16, 1980.
19. Reiz, S., Balfours, E., Freidman, A., et al. Acta Anaesthesiol. Scand. 25:103-10, 1981.
20. Reiz, S., Balfours, E., Haggmark, S., et al. Acta Anaesthesiol. Scand. 25:286-92, 1981.
21. Reiz, S., Balfours, E., Gustavsson, B., et al. Acta Anaesthesiol. Scand. 26:133-8, 1982.
22. Reiz, S., Balfours, E., Sorensen, M.B., et al. Anesthesiology 59:91-7, 1983.
23. Rydval, A., Haggmark, S., Nyhman, H., Reiz, S.: Acta Anaesthesiol Scand. 28:690-5, 1984.

CARDIOVASCULAR EFFECTS OF ISOFLURANE

P. FOËX

Isoflurane appears to possess several advantages over other halogenated anaesthetics in common use. Cardiac function is better maintained, ventricular arrhythmias are less likely to occur, profound muscle relaxation can be obtained, and biodegradation of the isoflurane molecule is only minimal. However, some of the effects of isoflurane on the circulation, while advantageous in some groups of patients may be disadvantageous in others. The main concern has been the possibility of coronary "steal" in patients with coronary heart disease.

Effects of isoflurane on the myocardium.

Isoflurane, like all inhalation anaesthetic agents exerts a negative inotropic effect on the isolated heart muscle (1). At concentrations corresponding to 1 MAC, depression of the active force developed by heart papillary muscles is reduced by about 40% by isoflurane, halothane and enflurane. Depression is even more marked when the heart muscle has been taken from a failing heart (2). The negative inotropy of isoflurane may be due to altered calcium ion movements either into or within the myocyte resulting in a reduced availability of calcium ions to initiate the interaction between actin and myosin (3,4).

Effects of isoflurane on the circulation.

Dose-dependent depression of cardiac contractility has been observed in response to stepped increases in alveolar concentration of isoflurane. However it was of smaller magnitude than the depression noted during halothane or enflurane anaesthesia. In clinical practice, the negative inotropic effect of the inhalation anaesthetics may be masked by the positive inotropic effect of sympathetic activation. By themselves, the modern inhalation anaesthetics do not increase sympathetic activity (5). However, hypercarbia, hypoxia, acute blood loss, anaesthetic manoeuvres and surgical manipulations may cause sympathetic overactivity.

While isoflurane resembles halothane and enflurane in that it causes a dose-dependent reduction of myocardial performance, it differs from both by causing dose-dependent peripherhal vasodilatation. Over a wide range of concentrations, isoflurane does not decrease cardiac output and the reduction of arterial pressure is due mostly to vasodilatation (6,7). As beta-adrenergic receptor blockade exerts only little effect on the responses of the circulation to isoflurane (7), the maintenance of cardiac output is not a reflection of sympathetic activation.

Effects of isoflurane on the coronary circulation.

The effects of isoflurane on the coronary circulation differ markedly from those of halothane and enflurane. Increases in alveolar concentration of isoflurane cause slight increases in coronary blood flow (8,9,10), while increases in halothane or enflurane concentration cause dose-dependent reductions of coronary blood flow (11,12,13). As isoflurane decreases contractility and arterial pressure, it also reduces myocardial oxygen consumption. Local regulation of coronary blood flow should result in commensurate reductions in oxygen demand and coronary flow. The uncoupling of coronary blood flow (unchanged) and oxygen demand (reduced), suggests that isoflurane impairs the local regulation of coronary blood flow. Indeed, the administration of isoflurane causes a dose-dependent reduction in coronary vascular resistance (10). This is accompanied by a substantial reduction of the coronary flow reserve. At 1.5 MAC isoflurane, the vasodilatory reserve was found to be almost exhausted in the dog (8). The reduction of resistance occurs in the small intra-myocardial vessels and not in the large coronary arteries (14). This drug-induced "luxury" perfusion of the myocardium may be of little consequence in the normal heart. It may even be beneficial in increasing local myocardial oxygen tension. However, luxury perfusion of normal myocardium may be at the expense of areas of the heart supplied by narrowed coronary arteries when ischaemic heart disease is present.

Isoflurane and myocardial ischaemia.

In patients with ischaemic heart disease, Reiz and colleagues have demonstrated a coronary vasodilating action of isoflurane (15). However, a high proportion of the patients developed myocardial ischaemia during steady-state anaesthesia during which arterial pressure, and hence coronary perfusion pressure were markedly decreased. Because isoflurane causes dilatation of small and not large coronary arteries, it is similar to dipyridamole which is used to produce non-homogenous distribution of coronary blood flow as a method of detecting flow-limiting coronary stenoses (16). Thus, the ischaemia observed during isoflurane anaesthesia (10,15) has been interpreted as evidence of coronary "steal". This implies that isoflurane interferes with the normal autoregulation of the coronary circulation, that is the ability to vary coronary blood flow (at similar coronary perfusion pressures), in response to changing oxygen needs. If coronary steal is present, flow through normal coronary vessels would have to be in excess of tissue requirements, and the coronary vascular reserve would have to be impaired

(17). This has been shown to occur with the administration of isoflurane (8). Moreover, redistribution of coronary blood flow during isoflurane anaesthesia has recently been reported in animal models. Isoflurane was found to redistribute blood flow from collateral-dependent to normal myocardium in dogs in which the left anterior descending coronary artery had been gradually occluded (18). The maldistribution was particularly marked at the subendocardium and was associated with impaired regional wall motion. In a model involving critical constriction of coronary arteries, isoflurane caused greater depression of compromised than normal myocardium (10,18). This was accompanied by the development of abnormal patterns of wall motion evidenced by the appearance of akinesia, paradoxical systolic lengthening, and post-systolic shortening (10). Thus, isoflurane, like other vasodilators of the coronary arterioles, can cause maldistribution of coronary blood flow, despite the reduced oxygen demand.

The steal phenomenon can be explained by the pressure gradient across coronary stenoses which reduces the distal perfusion pressure. As the distal small vessels are already maximally dilated, the administration of an arteriolar dilator can only reduce resistance in the normal territories, so that compromised territories receive less blood. Thus isoflurane is a potentially harmful anaesthetic agents for patients suffering from coronary artery disease. However not all patients will exhibit ischaemia. Those with multiple coronary artery lesions are more at risk (19), particularly when the concentration of isoflurane is such that their arterial pressure is markedly reduced.

Notwhitstanding these observation, the margin of safety of isoflurane determined as the fatal/anaesthetic ratio (FAR) in the swine is approximately double that of halothane and is not reduced by major surgery or the presence of critical coronary artery stenosis (20). The apparent discrepancy between an adverse effect on myocardium with compromised blood supply and the lack of reduction of FAR may relate to the favorable effect of isoflurane on the diastolic properties of the left ventricle. At variance with halothane (21) and enflurane (22), isoflurane causes reductions in end-diastolic pressure and dimensions (23). The improved relaxation, may protect the myocardium, at least in the case of single coronary lesions.

While isoflurane may be dangerous in some groups of patients, it could be the agent of choice in patients with arterial hypertension in whom reduction of afterload is desirable. The favorable effect of isoflurane on the diastolic properties of the left ventricle may be useful in patients with left ventricular hypertrophy. Like many other anaesthetic agents, isoflurane exerts profound effects on the heart and the circulation. Its safe use must be based on the understanding of its properties, including systemic and coronary vasodilatation, and on adequate monitoring of the circulation.

References.

1 Shimosato, S. and Etsten, B.E. (1969). Effects of anesthetic drugs on the heart: a critical review of myocardial contractility and its relationship to hemodynamics. Clin.Anesth., **9/13**, 17-29

2 Kemmotsu O., Hashimoto Y., and Shimosato S. (1973). Inotropic effects of isoflurane on mechanics of contraction in isolated cat papillary muscles from normal and failing hearts. Anesthesiology, **39**, 470-477.

3 Lynch C., Vogel S., and Sperelakis N. (1981). Halothane depression of myocardial slow action potentials. Anesthesiology, **55**, 360-368.

4 Blanck J.J., and Thompson M. (1982). Enflurane and isoflurane stimulate calcium transport by cardiac sarcoplasmic reticulum. Anesth.Analg. **61**, 142-145.

5 Skovsted, P. and Price, H.L. (1972) The effects of ethrane on arterial pressure, preganglionic sympathetic activity and barostatic reflexes. Anesthesiology, **36**, 257.

6 Stevens, W.C., Cromwell, T.H., Halsey, M.J., Eger, E.I., Shakespear, T.M., and Bahlman, S.H. (1971). The cardiovascular effects of a new inhalation anesthetic, forane, in human volunteers at constant arterial carbon dioxide tension. Anesthesiology, **38**, 8.

7 Horan, B.F., Prys-Roberts, C., Roberts, J.E., Bennett, M.J. and Foëx, P. (1977). Haemodynamic responses to isoflurane anaesthesia and hypovolaemia in the dog, and their modification by propranolol. Br.J.Anaesth., **49**, 1179.

8 Cutfield, G.R., Francis, C.M., Foëx, P., Ryder, W.A. and Jones, L.A. (1984). Isoflurane anaesthesia and coronary vascular reserve. Br.J.Anaesth., **56**, 1287P.

9 Priebe, H-J. (1987). Differential effects of isoflurane on regional right and left ventricular performances and on coronary, systemic and pulmonary hemodynamics in the dog. Anesthesiology, **66**, 262-272.

10 Priebe,H-J., and Foëx,P.(1987) Isoflurane causes regional myocardial dysfunction in dogs with critical coronary artery stenoses. Anesthesiology, **66**, 293-300.

11 Francis, C.M., Foëx, P., Lowenstein, E., Glazebrook, C.W., Davies, W.L., Ryder, W.A. and Jones, L.A. (1982). Interaction between regional myocardial ischaemia and left ventricular performance under halothane anaesthesia. Br.J.Anaesth., **54**, 965-980

12 Merin,R.G., Kumazawa,T., and Luka,N.L. (1976). Myocardial function and metabolism in the conscious dog and during halothane anesthesia. Anesthesiology, **44**, 402-411.

13 Merin,R.G. (1981). Are the myocardial and metabolic effects of isoflurane really different from those of halothane and enflurane ? Anesthesiology, **55**, 398-408.

14 Sill J.C., Bove A.A., Nugent M., Blaise G.A., Dewey J.D., and Gaban C. (1987). Effects of isoflurane on coronary arteries and coronary arterioles in the intact dog. Anesthesiology, **66**, 273-279.

15 Reiz S., Bolfors E., Sorensen M.B., Ariola S.jr., Friedman A., and Truedson H. (1983). Isoflurane - a powerful coronary vasodilator in patients with coronary artery disease. Anesthesiology, **59**, 91-97.

16 Brown B.G., Bolson,E.L., and Dodge,H.T. (1984). Dynamic mechanisms in human coronary stenosis. Circulation, **70**, 917-922.

17 Cohen M.V. (1982). Coronary steal in awake dog: a real phenomenon. Cardiovasc.Res., **16**, 339-349.

18 Buffington C.W., Romson J.L., Levine A., Duttlinger N.C., and Huang A.H. (1987). Isoflurane induces coronary steal in a canine model of chronic coronary occlusion. Anesthesiology, **66**, 280-292.

19 Becker,L.C. (1987). Is isoflurane dangerous for patients with coronary artery disease ? Anesthesiology, **66**, 259-261.

20 Roberts,S.L., Gilbert,M., and Tinker J.H.(1987). Isoflurane has a greater margin of safety than halothane in the swine with and without major surgery or critical coronary stenosis. Anesth.Analg., **66**, 485-491.

21 Doyle, R.L., Foëx, P., Ryder, W.A. and Jones, L.A. (1984). Effect of halothane on left ventricular relaxation. Br.J.Anaesth., **56**, 1286P.

22 Cutfield, G.R., Francis, C.M., Foëx, P., Ryder, W.A. and Jones, L.A.(1982). Enflurane, critical coronary stenosis, and left ventricular diastolic relaxation. Br.J.Anaesth., **54**, 1140P.

23 Foëx, P. (1987). Volatile anaesthetics and heart failure. In: Inhalation Anaesthetics, New Aspects, K.Peter, B.R.Brown. E.Martin and O. Norlander, Eds. Springer-Verlag, Berlin, pp. 207-218.

ANESTHESIA FOR MAJOR VASCULAR SURGERY -- CURRENT CONCEPTS

NORMAN J. CLARK, MD

INTRODUCTION

Vascular surgery has become a clearly recognized surgical subspecialty. Innovative surgical techniques and refinements in critical care have led to improved operative results with a wide range of complex vascular operations. These advances necessitate an increasingly specialized focus by anesthesiologists on the unique challeges and special intraoperative requirements of vascular surgery.[1,2] The present discussion will provide an overview of some anesthetic considerations for major vascular surgery, which for practical purposes, will be limited to operations on the abdominal or descending thoracic aorta that require a temporary period of aortic crossclamping. The merit of a separate focus on aortic surgery becomes apparent when one realizes that the morbidity and mortality attending operations on this major vessel still exceed that of other types of abdominal or thoracic surgery (Table 1). Violation of a major body cavity, eviceration of bowel and extensive retroperitoneal dissection (abdominal aorta), or collapse of lung and one lung

TABLE 1. Aortic surgery -- operative mortality

Abdominal aortic aneurysm	
1. Elective	4-8%
2. Emergency	
a) with preoprative shock	65-100%
b) no preopertive shock	8-58%
Abdonimal aortic occlusive disease	2-4%
Thoracic aortic aneurysm or dissection	
Type I (arch included)	25-43%
Type II (ascending only)	4-5%
Type III (descending only)	35-40%
Thoracic aortic trauma	20-30%
Coarctation of thoracic aorta	< 1%

ventilation, (thoracic aorta), along with the unique cardiovascular stress of aortic crossclamping all add up to a severe physiologic trespass. The interaction of these factors with coexisting diseases that are prevalent in these patients undoubtedly contributes to the higher morbidity and mortality seen in major vascular surgery. The objective of the following discussion will be to define, whenever possible, those aspects of anesthetic management that may influence the overall risk of surgery on the abdominal and/or thoracic aorta.

ABDOMINAL AORTIC SURGERY

Definition of Preoperative Risk Factors

The two major abdominal aortic lesions amenable to surgical repair are 1) aneurysm and 2) atherosclerotic occlusion. The high prevelance of co-existing disease in patients presenting with these lesions is apparent in every reported series.[1,3] The consistency of this finding may be taken as strong circumstancial evidence of the role of co-existing disease in perioperative morbidity and mortality. For example, in 1977, Young, et al,[3] reported a four-fold greater incidence of perioperative myocardial infarction following abdominal aortic aneurysmectomy in patients with evidence of coronary artery disease (CAD) (by history or EKG) compared to those in whom this evidence of CAD was absent. Recently, investigators have sought to define more precisely some valid clinical risk factors for abdominal aortic surgery. These retrospective studies have employed sophisticated statistical techniques to establish and quantify the relationship of a given preoperative condition to morbid or lethal perioperative events.

1978 - Cooperman, et al:[4] These investigators used multivariate analysis and identified five preoperative risks factors that had highly significant individual association with post-operative cardiovascular complications by Chi-square testing. The authors then used a logit distribution and recursive regression techniques to weight each risk factor. They developed an equation with which one could prospectively estimate the likelihood of cardiovascular complications when one or more risk factors were presesnt.

The risk factors were 1) prior myocardial infarction (MI), 2) congestive heart failure (CHF), 3) cardiac dysrhythmia, 4) abnormal EKG, and 5) previous cerebrovascular accident (CVA).

1986 - Yeager, et al:[5] Using mutivariate analysis and a logistic regression model, these authors defined four risk factors that had highly significant association with morbid or fatal cardiovascular complications. These factors were 1) history of MI, 2) CHF, 3) abnormal EKG, and 4) angina pectoris.

The implication of these findings is only partially clear. It is clear that some effort should be made preoperatively to determine the presence and severity of CAD and CHF. What remains unsettled is how far beyond routine history and physical examination one should go in evaluating the individual patient. Routine preoperative coronary arteriography is employed by some.[6] However, this approach is not taken by others who question the appropriateness of subjecting each surgical candidate to the risk of this additional invasive procedure.[7] At present, it seems helpful (and not unreasonable) to evaluate vascular surgery patients with provocative cardiac stress testing combined with either thallium scanning or 2D-echocardiography to identify the occurance of angina and its associaton with abnormalities in ventricular function. Alternatively, one could just assume that every patient has CAD with limited cardiac reserve and treat accordingly.

Aortic Crossclamping -- Pathogensis and Management of the Cardiovascular Stress

The nature of the cardiac stress that results from crossclamping the aorta anywhere along its course is best understood by considering the left ventricle (LV) as a "muscle-pump" functionally coupled to the systemic arterial circulation.[8] Studies with isolated cardiac muscle have identified certain intrinsic properties of cardiac muscle. These include contractility, ie., the ability to shorten against a mechanical load, and a set of length-force-velocity relations that describe the extent and velocity of shortening over a range of different loading conditions (ie., different degrees of preload and afterload).[8] These properties are the principle determinants of the way the left ventricle responds to aortic crossclamping. When cardiac muscle fibers are joined together in the three-dimensional configuration of the LV (roughly approximated by an ellipse rotated around its long axis), their collective shortening and relaxation create the action of a compression pump. The output of this pump is described with displacement terms such as stroke volume (SV), stroke work, ejection function (EF), cardiac output, etc.[8] Preload, the passive end-diastolic prestretch of the average sarcomere is now determined by the dimensions of the LV at end-diastole, translated most usefully as left ventricular end-diastolic volume (LVEDV). Afterload, the force sustained by the muscle during shortening is now governed by the La Place relation (T=Pr) and is defined as systolic wall tension (tension = force/circumfrential length), or more correctly stress (stress = tension/wall thickness). Because the LV is coupled with the systemic arterial circulation, it's afterload has two determinants;[9] 1) the ventricular muscle load resulting from the dimensions of the LV at onset of systole (ie., radius in the La Place equation), and 2) the vascular load, a result of aortic input impedance to ejection that creates back pressure in the LV during systole (ie., pressure in the La Place equation).[9] Aortic input impedance is a complex function that accounts for vascular resistance and aortic compliance as well as refected pressure and flow waves.[10] However, Gersh, et al,[11] and others[10] have shown that systemic vascular resistance (SVR) is the dominant term here, accounting for over 90% of aortic input impedance under usual conditions. Crossclamping the aorta decreases the capacity of the arterial vascular bed, increases all components of aortic impedance, and creates an instantaneous rise in LV systolic wall stress (afterload), the magnitude of which is related to how high on the aorta the crossclamp is placed. Because of the inverse relation between afterload and shortening that is intrinsic to cardiac muscle, fiber shortening decreases in response to the afterload stress, and all indicies of LV pump function that reflect fiber shortening (SV, EF, etc.) are thereby reduced (Table 2).[12-14] Left ventricular end-systolic volume (LVESV) increases by the amount that SV decreases. This produces an increase in LVEDV, tending to perpetuate the component of afterload stress resulting from ventricular enlargement. However, this is partially offset by a decrease in venous return from vasculature below the crossclamp that tends to decrease LVEDV and readjust wall stress downward within a few cardiac cycles.[1] The relative prominence of these

Table 2. Hemodynamic Changes of Aortic Crossclamping and Release in Humans[1] (Percent Change)

	Abdominal Aorta Infrarenal		Thoracic Aorta Below L Subclavian Artery	
	Crossclamp	Release	Crossclamp	Shunt Open
CO (L/min)	↓16–21%	NC–↑16%	↓29%	↑16%
SV (ml/beat//m²)	↓15–20%	NC–↑13%	↓32%	↑13%
LVSWI (gm-m/M²)	↓18–↑22%	↓10–45%	↓11%	↓19%
MAP (mm Hg)	↑7–12%	↓6–35%	↑35%	↓28%
SVR (dynes-sec-cm.5)	↑33–36%	↓12–30%	↑88%	↓38%
CVP (mm Hg)	↓50–↑26%	NC–↓30%	↑64%	↓32%
MPAP (mm Hg)	↓11–↑26%	↓20%	↑43%	↓33%
PVR (dynes-sec-cm.5)	↑15–40%	↓5–22%	↑57%	↓36%
PCWP (mm Hg)	↓23–50%	↓12–28%	↑83%	↓41%

CO = cardiac output; SV = stroke volume; LVSWI = left ventricular stroke work index; MAP = mean arterial pressure; SVR = systemic vascular resistance; CVP = central venous pressure; MPAP = mean pulmonary artery pressure; PVR = pulmonary vascular resistance; PCWP = pulmonary capillary wedge pressure. (NC = no change)

opposing influences on LVEDV determines the net effect of crossclamping on LV wall stress. In many patients a significant and sustained increase in LV wall stress is produced and the associated increase in myocardial oxygen requirement (MVO_2) seriously alters the myocardial O_2 supply/demand ratio and sets the stage for myocardial ischemia and acute ischemic ventricular dysfunction. A vicious cycle is thus initiated, whereby wall stress and MVO_2 are further increased as a result of ischemic compromise of LV systolic pump function.

When aortic crossclamping causes systolic blood pressure to rise to $\geq$ 180 mm Hg, or whenever evidence of myocardial ischemia is detected, pharmacologic afterload reduction with short-acting vasodilators is appropriate. It seems prudent in this setting to interpret a rise in PAOP of $\geq$3 mm Hg after crossclamping as evidence of ischemic ventricular dysfunction (ie, a stiffer ventricle) unless simultaneous 2-D TEE images are available that demonstrate that the ventricle has simply enlarged and moved to a higher position on its diastolic compliance curve.

Either nitroprusside and nitroglycerin can be employed for afterload reduction after aortic crossclamping.[12,17] A number of investigators have presented evidence that favors the use of nitroglycerin in this setting. Using a xenon-133 washout technique to measure regional myocardial blood flow, Mann et al,[15] demonstrated in humans that nitroprusside could redistribute myocardial blood flow away from ischemic areas by dilating coronary resistance vessels. This potentially detrimental effect was not seen with nitroglycerin. Using radiolabled microsphere in a canine model, Hummel, et al,[16] has shown that nitroglycerin preserves normal transmural myocardial blood flow distribution favoring the subendocardium after crossclamping the abdominal aorta. Zaiden, et al,[17] demonstrated in humans that low dose nitroglycerin infusion during the period of aortic crossclamping not only prevents the progressive rise in vascular resistance and fall in cardiac output, but also restores myocardial contractility back toward normal.

A second major anesthetic concern related to aortic crossclamping is occasioned by the removal of the crossclamp after completing the final graft anastomosis. This event promptly opens the distal vasculature to reperfusion, decreases aortic impedance, and reduces LV afterload. In most respects, the hemodynamic changes following release of the corssclamp are the exact opposite of those broght about by crossclamping. Although vascular resistance and arterial blood pressure and invariably reduced, cardiac output may increase or decrease.[1,12,18] At this time, the direction and magnitude of the change in cardiac output are critically dependent on LV preload, as measured by LV filling pressure, or more precisely, filling volume (ie, LVEDV). In the past, the term "declamping shock" was used to describe severe arterial hypotension and systemic perfusion failure that could develop after unclamping the aorta, and which occasionally progressed to intractable shock and death! Hypovolemia and/or mycardial depression due to wash-in of acid metabolites from post-ischemic tissues or release of myocardial depressant factors have been invoked as causes of this adverse development. It is now known that central hypovolemia, resulting from blood pooling in the dilated, flaccid, post-ischemic vasculature below the crossclamping site, is the major cause of hypotension or shock following aortic unclamping. Reiz, et al,[18] and others have shown that aggressive fluid loading so as to boost cardiac performance to a position on the higher, flatter portion of the Frank-Starling curve, usually maintains adequate cardiac output and prevents hypotension after aortic unclamping.[1,18]

Monitoring Cardiac Function During Aortic Surgery; Transesophageal Echocardiography-vs-PA Catheter

Recently, considerable interest has been focused on transesophageal 2-dimensional echocardiography (2-D TEE) as a sensitive, continuous, and minimally invasive monitor of cardiac function in patients undergoing major surgery. Accumulating evidence indicates that during aortic surgery it provides a more accurate measure of the impact of aortic crossclamping on LV dimensions and systolic function.[13,14,19,20] Echocardiographic detection of segmental wall motion abnormalities (SWMAs) also provides evidence of regional myocardial ischemia that precedes ischemia-related changes in the EKG or pulmonary artery occlusion pressure (PAOP).[21]

1983 - Roizen, et al:[13,14] These authors report 2-D TEE evidence that the magnitude of LV afterload stress and resulting ventricular dilation increases as the crossclamp is placed more proximally (higher) on the aorta.(Table 3) The incidence of SWMAs also increases with more proximal crossclamping.

Table 3. Changes in cardiovascular variables (%) by2-D TEE after aortic crossclamping[13]

	Level of aortic crossclamp		
	IR	SR	SC
MAP	↑2	↑5	↑54
PAOP	↑0	↑10	↑38
LVEDA	↑9	↑2	↑28
LVESA	↑11	↑10	↑69
LVEF	↓3	↓10	↓38
% with new SWMAs	0	33	92
% with new MI	0	0	8

IR = infrarenal; SR = suprarenal but infraceliac; SC = supracelian; MAP = mean artierial pressure; PAOP = pulmonary artery occlusion pressure; LVEDA = left ventricular end-diastolic area; LVESA = left ventricular end-systolic area; LVEF = left ventricular ejection fraction; SWMAs = segmental wall motion abnormalities; MI = myocardial infarction

1985 - Smith, et al:[21] In fifty patients undergoing vascular surgery (n=24) or coronary artery bypass grafting (n=21), 2-D TEE proved a more sensitive indicator of myocardial ischemia. Twenty-four patients developed new SWMAs whereas only six demonstrated ischemic ST segment changes with 7-lead EKG monitoring.

These finding have stimulated considerable interest and some debate regarding the clinical role of 2-D TEE. Should it become a routine monitor used in conjunction with the pulmonary artery catheter (PAC)? Should it replace the PAC in patients undergoing major surgery? Beaupre, et al,[22] have presented the somewhat disquieting evidence of frequent disparity between PAOP and left ventricular end-diastolic area (LVEDA) by 2-D TEE in patients undergoing major surgery including aortic reconstruction.[22] Linear regression of PAOP against LVEDA produced a correlation coefficient of <0.3 in 77% of these patients. In half the patients, occasions in which PAOP and LVEDA moved in opposite directions were observed. The authors invoked frequent intraoperative changes in LV compliance as an explanation for their findings.[22]

It is apparent from these results that if the PAC is used only to measure PAOP, and if inferences about LV function and preload are then drawn from this measurement, the information obtained will frequently be misleading. However, when most efficiently used, the PAC can provide considerably more information about cardiovascular function than PAOP alone. The PAC enables one to make repeated thermodilution cardiac output determinations, with which other hemodynamic indicies may be derived, and to measure mixed venous oxygen tension (Mv PO_2) or saturation (Sv O_2). The latter may be measured intermittentley, or with special fiberoptic catheters, continuously. The usefulness of this information and the role of the PAC in major vascular surgery has recently been reviewed.[23]

Conclusive evidence that use of the PAC favorably alters outcome in vascular surgery is lacking. Nevertheless, there appears to be a consensus in anesthesia and surgical literature that the PAC improves management of the patient undergoing major vascular surgery, and most anesthesiologists (including this author) are not ready to abandon its use. Transesophageal echocardiography requires fairly expensive equipment and requires a new set of pattern recognition skills to interpret the image it produces. Althrough few would question the value of the information obtained, at the present, the cost-vs-benefit issue remains unsettled with this monitor.

Anesthetic Management

General anesthesia using inhalational agents, intravenous agents, or both, as well as regional (continuous epidural) anesthesia have all been used successfully for major vascular surgery. Many anesthesiologists have taken the view that the particular agent or technique is immaterial, and it is rather the skill of the anesthesiologist that is crucial to successful outcome. This concept is supported by the findings of Bartkowski, et al,[24] of no significant differences in hemodynamic events or outcome among patients anesthetized with halothane-N_2O enflurane-N_2O, or morphine-N_2O for major vascular surgery. Cunningham, et al,[25] reported success with epidural block as a supplement to light general anesthesia. They observed no complications of epidural catheter placement even though each patient was given 3000 units of heparin intraoperatively. Others have shown that epidural blockade increases aortic graft blood flow acutely,[26] although long term effect on graft patency has not been demonstrated.

While few would dispute the requirement for skillful anesthetic management, recent evidence indicates that selection of particular anesthetic agents of techniques may also be of importance.

> 1986-Benefiel, et al:[27] These authors studied 100 patients randomly assigned to receive either isoflurane or sufentanil as a maintenance anesthetic during abdominal or thoraco-abdominal aortic reconstruction. Isoflurane anesthesia was associated with a four-fold greater incidence of post-operative renal insufficiency and a three-fold greater incidence of postoperative congestive heart failure compared to sufentanil anesthesia (Table 4). This is the first study to demonstrate major difference in perioperative morbidity between two anesthetic techniques for major vascular surgery.

Table 4. Number of post operative complications after major vascular surgery with isoflurane or sufentanil anesthesia

	Isoflurane (n=50)	Sufentanil (n=46)
Renal insufficiency	16*	4
Congestive heart failure	13*	4
Prolonged ventilation	9	4
Renal failure	3	1
Stroke	2	0
Myocardial infarction	0	1

*$P \leq 0.05$ by 2-tailed Fisher's exact test for difference from sufentanil

1987-Yeager, et al:[28] Perioperative morbidity and mortality were compared in 53 patients undergoing a variety of major surgical procedures, including major vascular surgery (n=22). By random assignment, 28 recieved epidural blockade as a supplement to light general anesthesia, and 25 receieved a "conventional" general anesthetic (balanced anesthesia or high dose fentanyl). Postoperative analgesia was provided through the epidural catheter (local anesthetics and/or narcotics) in the first group and with parenteral narcotics in the second group. The incidence of postoperative CHF, total complication rate and intensity, and cost of hospital stay were all significantly lower in the group managed with the epidural catheter.

It remains to be seen whether the results of these studies are reproducible by other investigators. Nevertheless, these results suggest that choice of anesthetic agent or technique may not be a trivial matter. It is interesting that Riez, et al,[29] first observed the isoflurane induced "coronary steal" phenomena in patients undergoing major vascular surgery. Whether an isoflurane-mediated "coronary steal" contributed to the differences in postoperative CHF observed by Benefiel, et al, is not known.

DESCENDING THORACIC AORTA

The major surgical lesions of the descending thoracic aorta include 1) coarctation, 2) dissection, ie., DeBakey type III, and 3) aneurysm. Chest trauma may also lacerate or rupture the aorta, or initiate a dissection that requires surgical repair. Although greater heterogeneity of age and physical status is seen in the presenting population, a high prevelance of coexisting disease is again encountered in those with aneurysm or dissection. The extent to which coexisting disease influences operative outcome is less clearly defined here than with abdominal aortic surgery. The principle causes of death following descending thoracic aortic aneurysmectomy in one large series were hemorrhage (29%), cardiac events (26%), and multi-organ system failure (22%).[30]

Surgical considerations include a decision as to whether left heart bypass or a heparin coated shunt will be employed to decompress the LV and perfuse the distal aorta during the period of aortic crossclamping. Although the shunt has become popular because it avoids the requirement for systemic heparinization, some surgeons proceed without any mechanical adjuncts to bypass the crossclamped segment of aorta. When this is the case, sodium nitroprusside (SNP), or less commonly, trimethophan, is administered to pharmacologically decompress the LV and proximal aorta during crossclamping.[31]

Besides anticipation of major blood loss and preparation for rapid transfusion, anesthetic considerations include 1) endobronchial intubation and use of one-lung ventilation, 2) application of invasive cardiovascular monitors, 3) adapting other monitoring devices to the constraints of the lateral decubitus position and requirements of one-lung ventilation, and 4) administration of a vasodilation such as SNP, when necessary for LV afterload reduction during aortic crossclamping. The relative merits of particular anesthetic agents or techniques have not been clearly defined. Data from animal studies indicate that potent inhalational anesthetics inhibit hypoxic pulmonary vasoconstriction (HPV), and could thereby increase shunting during one-lung ventilation. This is apparently not a clinical problem and their administration to patients undergoing one-lung ventilation does not impair oxygenation.[32]

Crossclamping the Descending Thoracic Aorta

Crossclamping the thoracic aorta just below the left subclavian artery produces a dramatic rise in aortic input impedance[9] and imposes a severe afterload stress on the LV.[9,33] Without immediate mechanical or pharmacologic afterload reduction, the markedly elevated systolic pressure and wall stress in the LV can lead to rapid decline in ventricular ejection, acute dilation and failure of the LV, mitral valve incompetance, frank pulmonary edema, and occasionally, fatal ventricular fibrillation.[1] Thoracic aortic crossclamping also markedly decreased spinal cord perfusion pressure and blood flow below the clamp.[34-36] Reductions in measured spinal cord blood flow of 84-97% have been reported. Since paraplegia is a most unwelcome and disturbingly frequent complication of operations on the descending thoracic aorta,[30,37] considerable effort has been directed to defining those surgical or anesthetic maneurvers that might influence the risk of this complication. Recently, attention has centered on the intraoperative use of somatosensory evoked potentials (SSEPs) to monitor spinal cord integrity, and on the relative advantages of mechanical adjuncts (shunts, partial bypass, etc.) for perfusing the distal aorta and reducing LV aftertload compared with pharmacologic afterload reduction alone.

Spinal Cord Injury and Spinal Cord Monitoring with Somatosensory Evoked Potentials (SSEPs)

Ischemic injury to the spinal cord complicates surgery on the descending thoracic aorta with a reported indicence of 1-10%.[38] The blood supply to the spinal cord, carried by the two posterior spinal arteries and one anterior spinal artery, is derived from radicular branches of extraspinal segmental arteries.[37] The level at which these segmental arteries send branches into the cord is quite variable. In particular, the large arteria radicularis magna anterior (artery of Adamkiewicz) which supplies a major portion of the lower anterior cord, originates between T_9 and T_{12} in 75% of cases, between T_5-T_8 in 15%, and at L_1 or L_2 in 10% of cases.[37] Ligation or disruption of this important supply vessel during resection of the diseased aortic segment can readily lead to ischemic cord injury. The clinical manisfestations of this injury are indistinguishable from the classical anterior spinal artery syndrome[37] and includes paraplegia, incontinence of bowel and bladder, loss of pain and temperature sensation, but preservation of vibratory and proprioceptive sensation. The pathogenesis of the cord injury is probably multi-factoral. Proposed mechanisms or contributory factors include 1) permanent interruption of critical supply vessels, 2) increased cerebrospinal fluid (CSF) pressure resulting from increased cerebral blood volume and flow following crossclamping, and 3) prolonged duration of aortic crossclamping resulting in insufficient spinal cord perfusion pressure below the clamp.[38] It has been suggested that CSF pressure exceeding aortic blood pressure below the crossclamp can "tamponade" spinal cord blood supply during crossclamping.[39,40] The use of mechanical adjuncts for perfusing the distal aorta during crossclamping has not proved successful in preventing ischemic spinal cord injury (or even reducing its incidence). Because of this, and because the anatomy of spinal cord blood supply is unpredictable in the individual patient, some means of continuously monitoring spinal cord function intraoperatively has been sought. Somatosensory evoked potentials (SSEPs) have shown some promise in this regard.

1982 - Cunningham, et al:[38] These investigators described three different type of response of SSEPs to crossclamping the descending thoracic aorta just below the left subclavian artery. Type 1 response consisted of a decrease in amplitude and increase in latency that began 3-4 minutes after crossclamping and progressed to complete flattening of the SSEP signal by 8-9 minutes. This response was associated with aortic blood pressures $\leq$ 25 mm Hg below the crossclamp and indicated loss of adequate perfusion to the distal cord. Type II response involved preservation of the baseline (pre-clamp) SSEP signal throughout the crossclamp period and was associated with blood pressures of 60-70 mm Hg below the clamp. This response was obtained when a shunt or bypass was used electively during crossclamping or in patient where "self-shunting" through physiologic collaterals occured. Type III response consisted of a delayed loss of the SSEP signal that was temporally related to ligation or surgical interruption of "critical intercostals" which were the source of important radicular branches to the cord. The authors proposed that recognition of these responses could guide intraoperative management. For example, type I response would indicate the need to utilize a shunt or bypass if crossclamping time were anticipated to exceed 30 minutes; type III response would indicate the need to surgically re-implant the critical vessels that had been interrupted.

Ischemic cord injury during aortic surgery primarily involves the anterior cord. Because SSEPs are conducted via the posterior columns of the cord it is perhaps inevitable that "false normal" SSEP signals will occur. One such case in a 55 year old male undergoing thoracic aortic surgery has been reported.[41] Other instances of postoperative paraplegia in patients in whom intraoperative SSEP signals remained normal, have been reported. These reports have been rare and it is not unreasonable to expect that use of SSEP monitoring to guide operative management, as outlined by Cunningham, et al,[38] may ultimately bring about a reduction in the incidence of paraplegia following aortic surgery. So far, the efficacy of this approach has not been evaluated prospectively.

Intraspinal Pressure and the use of Nitroprusside During Thoracic Aortic Surgery

The rise in proximal aortic blood pressure produced by crossclamping the thoracic aorta is transmitted to the cerebral circulation where it may exceed the upper limit of cerebral autoregulation.[35,39,40] An increase in cerebral blood volume and intracranial pressure (ICP) results. The rise in ICP is transmitted down the column of spinal fluid raising spinal fluid pressure around the spinal cord. The increase of CSF pressure following thoracic aortic crossclamping has been recorded in dogs[35,39] and in humans,[40] and can be measured in the cysterna magna,[39] or in the lumbar subarachnoid space.[35,40] The elevated CSF pressure may exceed blood pressure in the vasculature below the crossclamp and therby exacerbate the risk of spinal cord injury by "tamponading" spinal cord blood flow.[39,40]

Administration of nitroprusside has been shown to augment the rise in CSF pressure produced by aortic crossclamping[35,40] and to further decrease spinal cord perfusion pressure and spinal cord blood flow below the crossclamp.[34-36] Whether use of this drug has any influence on the incidence of ischemic spinal cord injury is not known. It has also been suggested the nitroprusside might improve spinal cord perfusion by lowering right artrial pressure and fascilitating venous drainage from the spinal cord,[42] although this hypothesis also lacks experimental verification. At the present time it is appropriate to only recommend caution in the use of nitroprusside and to give proper attention to other important details of anesthetic management, such as careful patient positioning so as to avoid venous (esp. jugular) outflow obstruction and avoidance of hypercarbia.

REFERENCES

1. Clark, N.J. and Stanley, T.H. In: Anesthesia 2nd Ed. (Ed. Miller, R.D.) New York, Churchill Livingston, pp. 1519-1562. 1986.

2. Florence, A.M. In: General Anaesthesia 4th Ed. (Eds. T.C. Gray, J.F. Nunn, and J.E. Utting) London, Butterworths, 1980, pp 1307-1323.

3. Young, A.E., Sandberg, G.W. and Couch, N.P. Am. J. Surg. 134: 585-590, 1977.

4. Cooperman, M., Pflug B., Martin, E.W., et al. Surgery 84:505-509, 1978.

5. Yeager, R.A., Weigel, R.M., Murphy, E.S., et al. Arch. Surg. 121:278-281, 1986.

6. Hertzer, N.R., Young, J.R., Kramer, J.R., et al. Arch. Surg. 114:1336-1344, 1979.

7. Brown, O.W., Hollier, L.H. and Pairolero, P.C. Arch. Surg. 116:1484-1488, 1981.

8. Weber, K.T. and Janicki, J.S. Am. Heart J. 98:371-384, 1979.

9. Covell, J.W., Pouleur, H., and Ross, J. Jr. Fed. Proc. 39:202-207, 1980.

10. Milnor, W.R. Circ. Res. 36:565-570, 1975.

11. Gersh, B.J., Prys-Roberts, C., Reuben, S.R., and Schultz, D.L. Brit. J. Anesth. 44:767-774, 1972.

12. Silverstein, P.R., Caldera, D.L., Cullen, D.J., et al. Anesthesiology 50:462-466, 1979.

13. Roizen, M.F., Beaupre, P.N., and Alpert, R.A. J. of Vasc. Surg. 1:300-305, 1984.

14. Roizen, M.F., Alpert, R.A., Beaupre, P.N., et al. Anesthesiology 59:A163, 1983.

15. Mann, T., Cohn, P.F., Holman, B.L., Green, L.H., Markis, J.E., Phillips, D.A. Circulation 57:(4)732-738 1978.

16. Hummel, B.W., Raess, D.H., Gewertz, B.L., Wheeler, H.T., Fry, W.J. Surgery 92:(2)159-166 1982.

17. Zaidan, J.R., Guffin, A.V., Perdue, G., Smith, R., McNeill, D.C., Arch. Surg. 117:1285-1288, 1982.

18. Reiz, S., Peter, T., Rais, O. Acta. Anaesth. Scand. 23:579-586 1979.

19. Roizen, M.F., Kremer, P., and Cahalan, M. Anesthesiology 57:A154, 1982.

20. Calahan, M.K., Kremer, P., Schiller, N.B., et al. Anesthesiology 57:A153, 1982.

21. Smith, J.S., Cahalan, M.K., Benefiel, D.J., et al. Circulation 72:1015-1021, 1975.

22. Beapre, P.N., Cahalan, M.K., Kremer, P.F., et al. Anesthesiology 59:A3, 1983.

23. Pace, N.L. In: Anesthesia for Vascular Surgery (ed. M. Roizen) New York, Churchill Livingston (in press).

24. Bartkowski, R.R., Aukburg, S.J., Greenhow, D.E. et al. Anesthesiology 51:S136, 1979.

25. Cunningham, F.O., Egan, J.M. and Inahara, T. The Amer. J. of Surg. 138:624-627, 1980.

26. Cousins, M.J. and Wright, C.J. Surg. Gynecol. and Obstet. July, 59-64, 1971.

27. Benefiel, D.J., Roizen, M.F., Lampe, G.H. et al. Anesthesiology 65:A516, 1986.

28. Yeager, M.P., Glass, D.D., Neff, R.K., and Brinck-Johnsen T. Anesthesiology 66:729-736, 1987.

29. Reiz, S., Balfors, E., Sorensen, M.B. et al. Anesthesiology 59:91-97, 1983.

30. Livesay, J.J., Cooler, D.A., Ventemiglia, R.A. et al. Ann. Thorac. Surg. 39:37-45, 1985

31. Shenaq, S.A., Chelly, J.E., Karlberg, H. Cohen E., Crawford E.S. Circulation 70(suppl 1), 1984.

32. Rogers, S.N., Benumof J.L. Anesth. Analg. 64:946-954, 1985.

33. Kouchoukos, N.T., Lell, W.A., Karp, R.B., Samuelson, P.N. Surgery 85:(1)25-30, 1979.

34. Gelman, S., Reves, J.G., Fowler, K., Samuelson, P.N., Lell, W.A., Smith, L.R. J. Thorac. Cardiovasc. Surg. 85:287-291, 1983.

35. Nugent, M., Kaye, M.P., McGoon, D.C., Anesthesiology 61:A68, 1984.

36. Kozody, R., Kehler, C.H., Duke, P.C., Parrott, J., Palahniuk, R.J., Wade, J.G. Anesthesiolgy 63:A47, 1985.

37. Costello, T.G., Fisher, A. Anaesthesia 38:230-236, 1983.

38. Cunningham, J.N., Laschinger, J.C., Merkin, H.A., Nathan, I.M., Colvin, S., Ransohoff, J., Spencer, F.C. Ann. Surg. 196:(3)285-296, 1982.

39. Blaisdell, F.W., Cooley, D.A. Surgery 51:(3)351-355, 1962.

40. Berendes, J.N., Bredee, J.J., Schipperheyn, J.J., Mashhour, Y.A.S. Circulation 66(suppl I)I-112-I-116, 1982.

41. Takaki, A., Okumura, F. Anesthesiology 63:(6)700-703, 1985.

42. Wadouh, F., Linemanm, E., Arndt, C.F. et al. J. Thorac. Cardiovasc. Surg. 88:1-10, 1984.

REVERSAL OF NEUROMUSCULAR BLOCKADE: CHANGING CONCEPTS

J. J. SAVARESE, M.D.

The philosophy of reversal of long-acting nondepolarizers is unchanged. The relatively long elimination half-lives (2-3 hours) of these drugs indicates that antagonism of residual block will nearly always be necessary.

Several recent studies have shown that antagonism of very deep block, where only one twitch in the train-of-four response may be visible, does require at least 15-30 minutes for achievement of maximum effect. In these cases, antagonism is sometimes incomplete, with train-of-four values reaching only 50-60 percent. The most effective antagonist in these situations is neostigmine in high dosage (0.06-0.08 mg/kg), together with an appropriate amount of atropine or glycopyrrolate.

Kopman has recently studied antagonism of deep block following long (>2 hrs) infusions of atracurium, vecuronium, and pancuronium (ref. 1). The relative "ease" of antagonism was related to the half-life of the relaxants, with atracurium showing the most rapid and consistent pattern of reversal, followed by vecuronium and pancuronium in that order. This study points out a novel concept: during "reversal," recovery from nondepolarizing block is simply being accelerated. The speed of reversal, therefore, especially if measured to completion of recovery (i.e. train-of-four value of greater than 70 percent) is influenced by the rate of spontaneous recovery of the drug, which in turn is reflected in the elimination half-life.

In clinical practice, this means that the chances of spontaneous recovery at the end of a procedure are greatest when atracurium is used as the relaxant.

Reversal may be viewed in another way: if reversal takes place at 25 percent twitch height, then speed of recovery to an end-point such as 95 percent twitch height may be compared during reversal or during spontaneous recovery. The data may be expressed as comparative 25-95 percent intervals. For atracurium, this interval is typically

20-25 minutes during spontaneous recovery. During induced recovery (reversal) with neostigmine (0.06 mg/kg), the interval is about 8 minutes (ref. 2), a difference of about 15 minutes. Therefore, reversal of atracurium block at 25 percent twitch height "saves" about 15 min. Comparative data for long-acting relaxants and the short-acting drug BW B1090U (mivacurium) are given in Table 1.

Table 1. 25-95 percent Intervals (min)

Drug	Spontaneous Recovery	Reversal	Time Saved (min)
Long-Acting Agents	60 - 120 (approx.)	8 - 10	50 - 110
Intermediate-Acting Drugs (Atracurium, Vecuronium)	20 - 40	8	10 - 30
Short-Acting Drugs (BW B1090U)	10	6	4

Inspection of Table 1 suggests that since the time "saved" by reversal of the short-acting drug BW B1090U (mivacurium) is only 4 min, in most cases administration of anticholinesterases may be superfluous (ref. 3). Reversal of the intermediate-acting drugs would save enough time to suggest that reversal might be beneficial to O.R. turnover, but nevertheless, in many carefully monitored cases, spontaneous recovery might be achieved if sufficient time were allowed. In my opinion, the philosophy of reversal of the intermediate-duration relaxants is "intermediate" as well: reversal should be undertaken on indication rather than in every case, especially during administration of atracurium, where the half-life is very short (20 min) and the metabolites have no effect on neuromuscular transmission.

One of the advantages of the newer drugs is the narrowing of the "time window" during which a drug interaction may occur, e.g., in the recovery room, with an antibiotic or antiarrhythmic agent. This time window approximates three half-lives of drug and equals about 60 minutes with atracurium, compared with six hours for long-acting drugs. It might be as little as 20 to 30 minutes after the short-acting drug BW B1090U, whose half-life may be as brief as eight to ten minutes. BW B1090U might very well dictate a change in attitude regarding reversal. In this case, reversal may seldom be required, assuming proper administration.

Accelerated reversal of nondepolarizing block has recently been reported by Abdulatif and Naguib (ref. 5, 6). In these studies, a "priming" dose of an anticholinesterase was followed 3 min later by the remainder of the drug. The "principle" here appears to be at least superficially similar to "priming" with nondepolarizing relaxants to accelerate onset of block.

REFERENCES

1. Kopman, A.F. Anesthesiology 65:572-578, 1986.
2. Basta, S.J., Ali, H.H., Savarese, J.J. et al. Anesth Analg 61: 723-729, 1982.
3. Savarese, J.J., Ali, H.H., Basta, S.J. et al. Anesthesiology 1988 (In press).
4. Savarese, J.J., Wastila, W.B. Seminars in Anesthesia 5:304-311, 1986.
5. Abdulatif, M., Naguib, M. Can Anaesth Soc J 33:723-728, 1986.
6. Naguib, M., Abdulatif, M., Absood, G.H. Anesthesiology 66:397-400, 1987.
7. Donati, F., McCarroll, S.M., Antzaka, C. et al. Anesthesiology 66:471-476, 1987.

PHARMACOLOGIC ANTAGONISTS IN ANESTHETIC PRACTICE

PETER L. BAILEY, M.D.

INTRODUCTION

Anesthesia is in many ways the clinical practice of pharmacology. Today's anesthesiologists are being asked to understand and use an increasingly diverse type and number of drugs. Ever since Langley discovered that a South American arrow poison paralyzed skeletal muscle, it has become increasingly evident that most drugs exert their effect through interactions with macromolecules that are now called receptors. Biologically, endogenous ligands (hormones, neurotransmitters) interact with receptors to maintain and regulate many aspects of body function.

Antagonist drugs, by strict definition, are compounds with high affinity and specificity for receptors that produce no effect via interaction at these sites except to block the action of agonists (endogenous ligands or exogenous substances). A more loose definition of antagonists includes agents that through receptor interactions may only partially block or modify the effect of endogenous ligands or exogenously administered compounds. Thus, calcium entry blockers and beta-adrenergic blockers produce antagonist effects that vary not only in proportion to their dose, but also with respect to the "state" of the cell, organ, system and body. Nalbuphine, on the other hand, is a partial-agonist/antagonist that can reverse or antagonize some opioid induced effects but in a limited yet complex fashion. Many antagonist compounds (Table 1), some old, some quite new, have diverse applications in anesthesia. A general overview will be accomplished in this section with detailed discussions on several newer antagonists.

ALPHA-ADRENERGIC RECEPTOR ANTAGONISTS

Ahlquist (1) first described alpha (α) and beta (β) receptors to delineate the effects of epinephrine, norepinephrine and isoproterenol and it is with these receptors that clinicians are most often familiar. Subsequent developments have revealed not only subtypes for these receptors

Table 1. Receptor antagonists used in anesthesia.

Receptor	Drug	Major Effect and Use
(Alpha Adrenergic)		
α_1	Prazosin	Reduces blood pressure/hypertension
α_1 and α_2	Phenoxybenzamine	Reduces blood pressure/pheochromocytoma
α_2	Yohimbine	Experimental
(Beta Adrenergic)		
β_1	Esmolol	Reduces heart rates, blood pressure and myocardial contractility
β_1 and β_2	Propranolol	Similar to esmolol
(Mixed)		
α_1 and β_1 and β_2		Labetolol Treat blood pressure and heart rate
(Cholinergic)		
Muscarnic	Atropine	Treat vagal related bradycardias
Nicotinic	Muscle relaxants	Muscle relaxation
(Serotonin)		
5-HT	Ketanserin	Treat serotonin induced effects
(Calcium Entry Blockers)		
	Nifedipine	Treat cardiac ischemia and high blood pressure
	Verapamil	Treat rapid supraventricular tachyarrythmias
	Diltiazam	Same as nifedipine and verapamil
(Dopamine)		
	Droperidol	Antinausea/antiemetic ? Potentiate hypoxic ventilary drive
(Benzodiazepine)		
	RO 15-1788 (Flumazenil)	Antagonize benzodiazepine sedation, amnesia, sleep and respiratory depression
(Opioid)		
	Naloxone	"Pure antagonist": reverses all agonist opioid effects
	Nalbuphine	Mixed partial agonist/antagonist: partial reversal of some opioid effects

but various agonists, antagonists, and even drugs with simultaneous but differing degrees of activity at more than one receptor. Thus alpha$_1$ (α_1) receptors are chiefly located at postsynaptic sites in smooth muscle and glands and alpha$_2$ (α_2) receptors mediate inhibition of neural release of norepinephrine at presynaptic sites. Alpha receptors also exist on platelets and, to a poorly defined degree, in the heart. Ischemia may increase α receptor population in the heart or enhance the arrhythmogenicity of α agonists (2). Beta$_1$ (β_1) receptors are predominately cardiac in nature and beta$_2$ (β_2) receptors are located in smooth muscle and gland cells, though both types of receptors are often found in the same tissues.

Prazosin (Minipress^R) is the most specific α_1 antagonist and is virtually devoid of α_2 antagonism. Its postsynaptic α_1 blockade in vascular beds is useful in the oral treatment of chronic hypertension. Its antihypertensive effect begins to decrease 8 to 12 hours after administration. Phenoxybenzamine (Dibenzyline^R) is known to clinicians who prepare patients with pheochromocytoma for surgery. It is antagonistic at α_1 and less so at α_2 receptors and binds to them irreversibly through a covalent bond. (After the surgical removal of hormone producing tumors in pheochromocytoma patients, exogenous norepinephrine infusions may be necessary to override this now unopposed α blockade). Phentolamine (Regitine^R) binds equally to α_1 and α_2 receptors. The α_2 antagonism enhances norepinephrine release and leads to increased inotropism and chronotropism and thus can worsen angina. Prazosin, because of its lack of α_2 antagonism rarely leads to tachycardia. Alpha$_2$ antagonism is experimentally produced by yohimbine. The clinical usefulness of such a type drug in man has not become apparent. Theoretically it could be of benefit in patients with idiopathic autonomic dysfunction. [Alpha$_2$ agonism with clonidine has on the other hand found several clinical applications, e.g., as an antihypertensive and premedicant to reduce anesthetic requirements (3)].

BETA-ADRENERGIC RECEPTOR ANTAGONISTS: ESMOLOL

Beta receptor antagonism is known to be helpful in treating supraventricular tachyarrhythmias (SVT), hypertension, cardiac ischemia, and, perhaps in reducing myocardial infarct size (4). In the perioperative period, β blockade has been shown to help stabilize hemodynamics during intubation and other stressful periods (5,6). Prior to esmolol, the long duration of action of available beta blockers and the risk of inducing or exacerbating hypotension, cardiac failure or bronchospasm represented real limitations in applying acute beta blockade therapy. Esmolol, a new, very short-acting cardioselective beta-adrenergic antagonist, permits β_1 blockade with little concomitant risk due to a rapid abatement of its effects, should they be deleterious, within 5-15 min when its infusion is stopped (7). Esmolol's onset of action is within 1 to 2 minutes. Its redistribution half-life is 2 minutes and its elimination half-life is 9 minutes. It is metabolized by esterases within red cells (not serum cholinesterase) and its clearance is 20 L/kg/hr (8).

Esmolol is usually prepared for administration by putting 5 g (2 ampules) in 500 cc (1% solution or 10 mg/ml). Infusions of 50-500 µg/kg/min rapidly produce serum levels that are therapeutic. Perioperative supraventricular tachyarrhythmias, especially those associated with endotracheal intubation and other stressful stimuli, are effectively treated with 50-500 µg/kg/min in numerous studies in man. In addition, 100-300 µg/kg/min has been shown to be safer in asthmatics in whom propranolol significantly increased airway resistance or induced bronchospasm. Tachycardias or rapid heart rates placing cardiac ischemic patients at risk can also be effectively treated with titrated infusions of 50-500 µg/kg/ min. Moderate hypertension can similarly be treated. Compared to nitroprusside, esmolol therapy will avoid increases in heart rate and maintain diastolic blood pressures at more desirable levels due to lesser decreases in systemic vascular resistance. In addition, arterial oxygen saturation does not decrease with esmolol as it does with nitroprusside (9), Table 2.

Table 2. Esmolol vs. nitroprusside.

	Significant Directional Changes After	
Parameter	Esmolol	Nitroprusside
Heart Rate	↓	↑
Blood Pressure		
Systolic	↓	↓
Diastolic	↓	↓
Cardiac Index	↓	↑
PaO2	→	↓
O_2 Saturation	→	↓

Clinicians should proceed with caution when using esmolol in patients at risk for congestive failure, significant hypotension, or bronchospastic disease. The signs and symptoms of hypoglycemia can be masked, and prior catecholamine depletion (reserpine therapy) may potentiate esmolol's effects, as may other drugs with myocardial depressant properties. Concomitant administration of analgesic doses of morphine can also lead to higher than expected esmolol serum concentrations. Esmolol can prolong the duration of succinylcholine-induced blockade by 5 to 8 minutes.

Esmolol offers the opportunity to apply "on-off" pharmacologic control of heart rates and blood pressures that endanger patients at risk for cardiac ischemia. However, the type of anesthesia, the degree of surgical stimulation, and the adrenergic state of the patient are all important clinical considerations that will mandate significant experience, judgment and skill when using esmolol.

MIXED ALPHA AND BETA-ADRENOCEPTOR ANTAGONISTS: LABETOLOL

Labetolol hydrochloride (Trandate^R, Normodyne^R) is a newly released, combined alpha- and beta-adrenoceptor blocker (10). Its beta antagonism is nonselective, though more potent at β_1 than at β_2 receptors, and its potency is approximately one-third that of propranolol. In addition, labetolol may possess mild β_2 agonist properties (intrinsic sympathomimetic activity)(11). Labetolol has alpha antagonist effects that are restricted to post-synaptic α_1 receptors. It is one-tenth as potent as phentolamine at these receptors. Overall labetolol's beta-blocking effects are approximately seven times greater than its actions at alpha receptors (12). Although available as an oral agent, this discussion will concentrate on its intravenous use.

Intravenous administration of labetolol produces a rapid onset (within minutes) of an anti-hypertensive effect that is proportional to the severity of the sympathetic drive: the more marked the hypertension (and tachycardia), the greater the reductions. Thus titration of 5-20 mg boluses, up to 250 mg, if needed, rarely produces overshoot and undesired hypotension or bradycardia. Since propranolol is not as effective in lowering blood pressure, labetolol's alpha blocking properties probably play an important role in its rapid antihypertensive effect.

After intravenous administration labetolol's effect peaks rapidly (5-15 min). Its distribution half-life is 6 min and it is 50% bound to plasma proteins. Its volume of distribution (steady state) is about 9 L/kg. Its clearance rate is 1-2 L/min and its elimination half-life is 3-7 hr. Renal failure apparently produces little increase in its duration of effect as it is mostly metabolized in the liver by conjugation to glucuronide metabolities that have very little activity themselves. Labetolol produces minimal decreases in hepatic blood flow and patients do not experience tachyphylaxis. Simultaneous medical therapy with cimetidine will increase its bioavailability (13).

Compared to traditional beta blockers, labetolol offers advantages when treating hypertensive patients, especially if cardiac failure is also a risk. Cardiac output is maintained near normal after labetolol (decreased with propranolol) left ventricular end-diastolic pressure decreases (can increase with propranolol), and systemic vascular resistance falls modestly (increases with propranolol). Heart rate decreases, but less so compared to propranolol. Compared to pure alpha-blocking or vasodilating antihypertensive compounds, labetolol therapy avoids the risk of reflex tachycardia (Table 3). Thus it is similar to pharmacologic combinations like propranolol and prazosin or propranolol and hydralazine (14).

Table 3. Resting hemodynamic effects of propranolol, prazosin and labetolol.

	Propranolol	Prazosin	Labetolol
Blood pressure	↓	↓	↓
Heart rate	↓↓	→↑	↓
Cardiac output	↓↓	→↑	→↓
Stroke volume	↓	↑	→↑
Systemic vascular resistance	↑	↓	↓
LVEDP	→↑	↓	→↓

(Adapted from Carter BL, ref. 13)

Rapid amelioration of perioperative hypertension can usually be obtained with two or three boluses of 10 to 20 mgs of labetolol. Immediate preoperative treatment shold be tempered by the fact that synergism with potent inhalation agents such as halothane exists. The cardiac depressant effects of any drug may be potentiated in the presence of labetolol, and vice versa. On the other hand, this author has used labetolol often during and immediately following anesthesia and has not yet experienced undesirable hypotension or bradycardia.

Although some evidence and authors suggest labetolol may be a safer beta-blocker in patients with bronchospastic disease (15), asthma can be exacerbated by labetolol and should probably be avoided in this patient population. Poor left-ventricular function or heart failure, as with other beta blockers, represent contraindications to the use of labetolol. In addition, reservations persist regarding the use of labetolol in obstetrical anesthesia despite low placental transfer because of inadequate fetal and newborn outcome studies. Postural hypotension, the most common adverse effect, can also occur with IV labetolol and one should observe for this effect especially in patients that ambulate soon after surgery.

Careful titration of labetolol in pediatric and geriatric patients as well as middle-aged adults should produce good results when treating hypertension. However, as always, when treating a sympathetic response during anesthesia and surgery, it behooves the clinician to make sure that such a response is not an important and appropriate homeostatic reflex to such stimuli as hypovolemia, hypoxia, hypercarbia, hypoglycemia, or light anesthesia, and that conditions such as allergic phenomenon, thyroid storm, and malignant hyperthermia do not exist. Once such conditions have been excluded, the anesthesiologist can assume excessive sympathetic drive exists and treat it directly with agents such as labetolol.

HISTAMINE ANTAGONISTS

Histamine contracts smooth muscle in the bronchi and gut (H_1 receptors) and relaxes smooth muscle in small blood vessels, especially terminal arterioles (H_1 and H_2 receptors) causing decreases in total peripheral resistance and systemic blood pressure. Possible constriction in large blood vessels may increase total peripheral resistance. Capillary leak and edema formation due to histamine are related to H_1 more than H_2 receptors. In the heart histamine directly increases the force of contraction, heart rate and automaticity (H_2 receptors), while decreasing A-V conduction (H_1 receptors). Thus diverse arrhythmias can be elicited by histamine. Reflex responses to the systemic and vascular effects of histamine may override its direct effects.

H_2 receptors predominate in the stomach. There, histamine, through its interaction with H_2 receptors increases the activity of adenylate cyclase in parietal cells leading to stimulation of the Hydrogen-Potassium ATPase pump, extrusion of protons, and a drop in the pH of gastric secretions. H_2 blockade decreases gastric volume and increases gastric pH during basal (fasting) secretion, nocturnal secretion and food stimulation.

The above description points to two of the more important indications for histamine antagonists in anesthesia. Philbin et al. (16) demonstrated that both H_1 and H_2 blockade was essential if the hemodynamic effects of histamine, released during a morphine induction, were to be maximally attenuated. Thus, preinduction treatment with cimetidine (4 mg/kg) and diphenhydramine (1 mg/kg) permitted a morphine induction with much less decrease in systemic vascular resistance and diastolic blood pressure than when no antagonist or just one antagonist was given. Some adverse effects of other histamine releasing drugs or drug reactions (e.g., protamine) may also be decreased by histamine antagonists.

Mendelson's clinical case descriptions detailing the consequences of aspiration (17), highlighted the importance of preventing this complication in obstetric patients. To this day, prophylaxis and prevention remains better than treatment and cure of aspiration in any patient population. The H_2 receptor antagonists, one of the most prescribed medications in North America, have also found a place in the anesthesiologist's pharmacy due to their ability to raise gastric pH (18,19) and decrease gastric volume (19) and presumably reduce the morbidity and mortality of aspiration. Thus it would appear logical to use H_2 antagonists in certain patient populations: trauma victims and other emergencies, patients with gastro-esophageal reflux and hiatal hernia, obese patients, obstetrical patients, outpatients, patients with intestinal obstruction, and perhaps cases where general anesthesia is to be delivered by mask. However, in addition to cost and a lack of trials proving a real reduction in morbidity and mortality with such an approach, other considerations may limit the use of these drugs, especially on any routine basis. Cimetidine, the first H_2 antagonist available in America, may produce some undesirable side effects. It can cause CNS depression, bradycardia with hemodynamic compromise upon rapid intravenous injection, and decrease hepatic clearance (either through decreased hepatic blood flow and/or decreased microsomal activity) of various drugs including warfarin, diazepam, phenytoin, theophylline, propranolol, and lidocaine. Airway reactivity in asthmatics may be exacerbated by H_2 antagonism as H_2 receptors may have a bronchiolar relaxing function (20). In addition, it should be recognized that the acidity of gastric contents already present is not altered by the administration of cimetidine, or the newer H_2 antagonist ranitidine. Rantidine offers advantages over cimetidine in that it causes fewer adverse reactions and drug interactions and lasts longer. However, other limiting considerations made above remain.

Cimetidine apparently works best when given the night before and the morning of surgery. Oral or intramuscular injection is preferable (300-400 mg) and its effects peak in 60-90 min and last 4 hr. The dosage for ranitidine is 50-100 mg IV or 150 mg po and its duration of effect is longer, up to 8 hr.

Other histamine antagonists familiar to clinicians include hydroxyzine (vistaril) and promethazine (phenergan).

BENZODIAZEPINE ANTAGONISM: FLUMAZENIL (RO 15-1788)

Specific benzodiazepine receptors were discovered in 1977 (21,22). They exist in highest concentration in the cerebral cortex but also in the hypothalamus, the cerebellum, the corpus striatum and the medulla. Benzodiazepines have anti-anxiety and anticonvulsant effects and produce sedation, amnesia, sleep, muscle relaxation and respiratory depression. The regional distribution of benzodiazepine receptors parallels that of gamma-aminobutyric acid (GABA) receptors but they are not one in the same. Their proximity, however, points to the biochemical mechanism of benzodiazepines: probably through an allosteric change in the GABA receptor complex, benzodiazepines increase the firing of synapses using GABA as a neurotransmitter. GABA is the major neuroinhibitory transmitter in the brain (it increases chloride ion conductance which hyperpolarizes cell membranes). Glycine appears to play the role of GABA in the spinal cord and brain stem and has similar interactions with benzodiazepines (Fig. 1).

Preoperative sedation with the numerous benzodiazepines available today is popular. Also, the introduction of midazolam has brought a benzodiazepine into the anesthesiologist's aramamentarium that has numerous advantages over diazepam for intravenous use in the operating room: it is water soluble, does not cause pain or a high incidence of phlebitis on injection, is more rapid acting, more potent, shorter acting and its duration of effect is less affected by age. Sedation with a benzodiazepine like midazolam during monitored anesthesia care or regional anesthesia helps provide patient comfort, light sleep, and amnesia. The ability to reverse the sedation at the end of surgery would offer several advantages: reversal of the respiratory depressant and sleep inducing effects of benzodiazepines, early discharge to and from recovery facilities and outpatient departments and better cooperation from a more lucid patient during recovery. In addition, anesthetic induction with midazolam, supplemented with moderate doses of fentanyl (2-5 μg/kg) is easily achieved. This technique supplemented with nitrous oxide might be useful if a wake-up test is

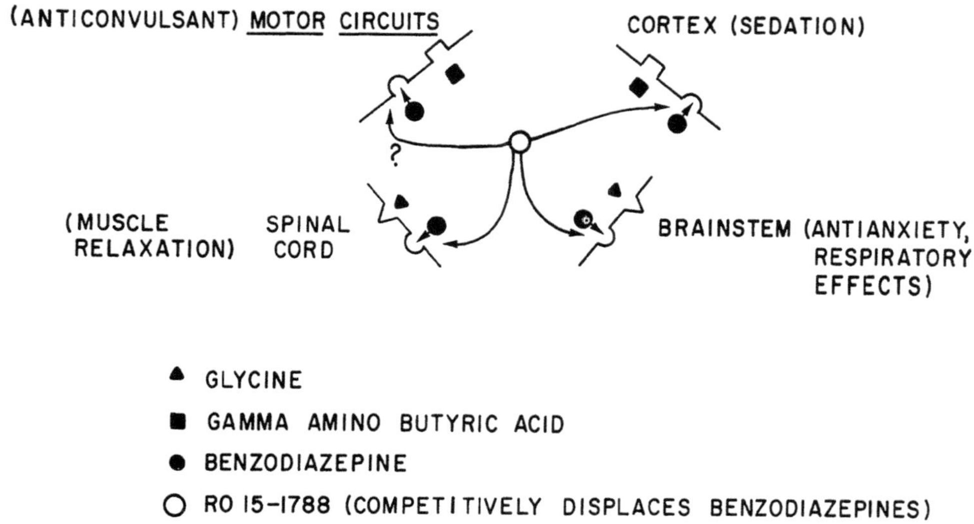

Fig. 1. Benzodiazepine effects: Mediated through GABA and glycine receptors.

required (e.g., Harrington rodding) or in other unique anesthetic circumstances. Other applications of a specific benzodiazepine antagonist include treatment of the overdose patient and reversal of the rare but frightening paradoxical reaction to benzodiazepine administration.

In the past, only stimulant drugs (e.g., theophyline, physostigmine) were available as nonspecific antagonists of benzodiazepines, and they produced erratic results. More recently through work on a series of imidazodiazepine compounds, a receptor specific antagonist with high affinity, RO 15-1788 (Flumazenil/Anexate) has been developed (23). Animal studies have demonstrated the safety and specificity of RO 15-1788 (23). Human studies have also documented its safety (24) and efficacy (25) and it has been in clinical use in Europe and Britain for several years.

Flumazenil, in either titrated doses (0.2 mg per min)(26) or intravenous boluses (10 mg)(25), has a rapid onset of effect (1-3 min). Pharmacokinetic data are scant (27,28) but the plasma half-life of flumazenil appears to be approximately 30 to 80 min with a volume of distribution of 1 L/kg, and a clearance of 1.14 L/min, and a duration of action of 1 to 3 hr. In the presence of large doses of benzodiazepines or long-acting agents, "renarcotization" may occur after reversal with flumazenil (25). In various studies, flumazenil reverses the sedation (25,26), respiratory depression (29), EMG (30), and cerebral depressant effects (31) of benzodiazepines. When injected alone flumazenil has little effect, although dizziness has been reported. Flumazenil does not appear to antagonize the anticonvulsant effects of benzodiazepines and may have some anticonvulsant activity on its own. Some patients do experience anxiety after reversal with this agent and benzodiazepine withdrawal can be precipitated by RO 15-1788. It has also been used successfully in reversing comatose states in patients overdosed with benzodiazepines (32). In a recently completed study at our institution flumazenil produced a rapid reversal of sedation without the hemodynamic alterations. Importantly, no other study has pointed to any significant hemodynamic changes associated with flumazenil antagonism of benzodiazepine mediated effects. In addition, improved arterial blood gases existed when patients received flumazenil after general anesthesia with flurazepam, fentanyl, pancuronium, N_2O and O_2 (33).

Thus it appears that flumazenil will provide anesthesiologists with a specific antagonist to reverse the potent amnesia and sleep inducing effects of midazolam and other benzodiazepines. It has few adverse effects, is rapid acting, and its major limitation will be its short duration of action, that depending upon numerous clinical factors (e.g., dose and type of benzodiazepine and dose of flumazenil used) may or may not be an important consideration. These and other elements of the use of RO 15-1788 will require further investigation and description.

NARCOTIC (OPIOID) ANTAGONISTS

From the beginning of this century to this day the use of narcotics in anesthesia has often been limited by respiratory depression and the possible subsequent morbidity (34). In spite of more than three decades of research a consistently effective opioid antagonist that is without adverse effects is not available.

In the 1950's, nalorphine (35) and levallorphan (36) were evaluated as narcotic antagonists and not found satisfactory (37). Naloxone held promise of being a superior narcotic antagonist when it was introduced in the 1960's, and it was. Initial enthusiasm, however, was tempered by clinical reports of serious adverse effects: hypertension (38,39,40), cerebral vascular accident (39), ventricular arrhythmias (41), pulmonary edema (42-45) and cardiac arrest and death (46) (Table 4). The value of case reports in this author's opinion is dubious at best. Confounding factors such as the concomitant administration of other drugs (e.g., physostigmine) (38), the possibility of other causes of ventilatory depression (e.g.,

Table 4. Reported severe complications following naloxone.

Author	Naloxone Dose (IV, mg)	Complication
Azar	0.4	HTN (270/140)
Estillo	0.4	HTN (260/140); CVA
Flacke	0.4	Pulmonary edema
Tanaka	0.4	HTN (340/150)
Andree	0.4	Cardiac arrest; death
	0.4	Cardiac arrest; death
Prough	0.1	Pulmonary edema
	0.2 (+0.3 IM)	Pulmonary edema
Michaelis	0.1	V TACH, V FIB
	0.4	V FIB
Partridge	0.08	Pulmonary edema
Taff	0.3	Pulmonary edema

laryngospasm), and the reported need for naloxone to antagonize quite small doses of fentanyl in large healthy young adults make drawing objective conclusions from such articles difficult if not at times misleading. In addition, the doses of naloxone most commonly used in these case reports (0.4 mg IV bolus in seven of twelve cases) are excessive and unnecessary (see below). Although naloxone can be used safely, the possibility of severe increases in HR and BP, pain and renarcotization do make naloxone far from ideal.

Most recently nalbuphine (Nubain®), a mixed agonist-antagonist opioid, has been evaluated as an alternative to naloxone for reversal of narcotic-induced respiratory depression (47-53). None of these reports compared nalbuphine with naloxone in a double-blind fashion. Some of these references report complications attributed to nalbuphine yet ask readers to accept clinical and pharmacologic scenarios that are not possible (53). Nonetheless, purported advantages of nalbuphine over naloxone have been the production of less hemodynamic change, adequate analgesia after reversal, and a duration of effect (3-5 hours) that lessens the chance for renarcotization compared to naloxone (duration of effect 30-90 min).

Nalbuphine has activity at mu as well as kappa opioid receptors. It has agonist properties at kappa receptors where it mediates analgesia and perhaps some mild respiratory depression. Nalubphine is either devoid of mu activity (antagonist) or possesses weak mu activity (partial agonist). It is not clear which is the case in man.

It is established that nalbuphine will not antagonize analgesic doses of opioid analgesics: the respiratory and analgesic effects of morphine, 15 mg IV, are in fact potentiated by attempted reversal with nalbuphine (54). However, this author and his colleagues believed nalbuphine to be superior to naloxone for the reversal of postoperative opioid-induced respiratory depression and performed a comparative double-blind clinical study. In that study (55), 90 patients received a mean dose of 25 μg/kg of fentanyl along with 60% N_2O and 40% O_2 and isoflurane, 0.1 to 1.0% to maintain blood pressure within 25% of control, for anesthesia lasting 3 ± 1 hr. Fentanyl was administered as 15 μg/kg over 2 min during induction and then 50 μg every 15 min. End-tidal CO_2 was maintained at 40 ± 2 mm Hg. Inadequate spontaneous ventilation at the end of anesthesia (T.V. < 4 ml/kg or RR < 8) was treated with naloxone .08 mg or nalbuphine 2.5 mg IV every 2 min until spontaneous ventilation was adequate and patients were extubated.

Only 60 of 90 patients required narcotic reversal attesting to the variability of the degree of respiratory depression after fentanyl. Patients reversed with naloxone required only one or two doses (.08 or .16 mg) 90% of the time and three doses (.24 mg) 10% of the time. Patients reversed with nalbuphine required one to three doses (2.5 to 7.5 mg) 90% of the time and a maximum of four doses (10 mg) 10% of the time. Both drugs produced similar, moderate increases in heart rate, blood pressures, and rendered respiratory rates and tidal volumes adequate. Arterial blood gas changes were similar in both groups (Table 5).

Analgesic requirements (administered as 2 mg boluses of morphine or 25 mg boluses of meperidine if patients complained of pain more than once in a 5-min period or complained of severe pain) were significantly less in patients antagonized with nalbuphine (Table 6). In addition, renarcotization occurred more often in patients reversed with naloxone (5 of 30) compared to nalbuphine (2 of 30) but this difference did not reach statistical significance.

Other reports (52) have at least anecdotally confirmed our belief that favorable results can be achieved when reversing narcotic depression with small doses of nalbuphine (2 to 3 mg) by intermittent bolus (every 2 to 3 min). Although small doses of naloxone or nalbuphine administered as narcotic antagonists may rarely produce serious adverse effects, we

Table 5. Arterial blood gases at the onset of spontaneous respiration and 30 and 60 min later (mean ± SD) after opioid antagonism with naloxone (Nx) or nalbuphine (Nb).

		Onset S.R.	30′	60′	Range
	pH	7.30±.09	7.33±.09	7.32±.06	
Nx	PCO_2 (mmHg)	49.2±9.5	43.9±9.4	42.5±9.5	(19-65)
	PaO_2 (mmHg)	209±88	128±53	102±63	
	pH	7.27±.06	7.32±.04	7.33±.03	
Nb	PaCO2 (mmHg)	50.2±8.7	43.2±5.2	42.5±4.3	(30-69)
	PaO_2 (mmHg)	183±80	120±52	84±45	

Table 6. Patients requiring analgesics in the recovery room after opioid antagonism with naloxone (Nx) or nalbuphine (Nb)

	Number	Percent
Nx	12/30	(40)
Nb	5/30*	(16.7)*

*P < 0.05 compared to Nx group (see text for details).

did not experience any in our study. Occasionally, the pain a postoperative patient experiences after antagonism is difficult to treat but this is uncommon. Contrary to the practice and belief of some anesthetists, this author has found that larger single doses of nalbuphine (10 to 20 mg) are more likely to produce adverse effects and pain. Caution should still be practiced in regards to narcotic antagonism:

1) avoid opioid antagonists in patients with cardiovascular disease, e.g., coronary artery disease, hypertension
2) avoid opioid overdose in healthy patients scheduled for routine

surgery where adequate return to consciousness and spontaneous ventilation and extubation are expected

3) allow adequate arterial carbon dioxide levels to develop and stimulate respiratory drive prior to narcotic antagonism

4) use small doses of naloxone or nalbuphine and wait 2 to 3 min ("real time") between doses

5) the use of opioid antagonists are rarely necessary and should not substitute for good anesthetic technique

The recent division of mu receptors into mu_1 and mu_2 with the suggestion that respiratory and analgesic effects can be separated via these two different receptor subtypes points toward a possible resolution of the "analgesia-without-respiratory depression" narcotic problem. As of yet, however, there is still no ideal pharmacologic answer on the horizon.

SEROTONIN ANTAGONISTS

Serotonin is predominantly located in the GI tract of man but is also found in systemically circulating platelets and in the brain. Serotonin or 5-hydroxytryptamine (5-HT) receptors are of at least three subtypes (56) and through these receptors serotonin mediates vascular constriction, bronchoconstriction, platelet aggregation and neuronal effects. Ketanserin has been the most widely investigated serotonin (5-HT_2) antagonist (57). Ketanserin, although still experimental in the United States, holds promise for treating various hypertensive states (e.g., following cardiopulmonary bypass), shock states (e.g., endotoxic), thrombotic processes, peripheral vascular diseases and sympathetic dystrophies (58). 5-HT_1 receptors mediate serotonin induced stimulation of adenylate cyclase, inhibition of neurotransmitter release and contraction in certain arterial systems (59). 5-HT_2 receptors are widely distributed in the peripheral nervous system and mediate many of serotonin's excitatory actions and influence nociception. Recently developed experimental antagonists and agonists of these 5-HT receptors are helping further define the therapeutic roles manipulation of serotonin receptors will play in the future.

CALCIUM ENTRY BLOCKERS (CEB)

It is not the purpose in this section to comprehensively review CEB's but to place them in the overall scheme of antagonist-type drugs. CEB's modulate the entrance of calcium either through voltage-dependent channels (depolarization of the cell membrane increases the probability of these channels opening) or similar receptor-operated channels (60). Although intracellular stores of calcium can also be released by stimulation of cell surface receptors by neurotransmitters or hormones, the mechanism is not well defined and will not be discussed here (61).

Voltage-dependent calcium channels (VDCC) are widely distributed in man and present in smooth, cardiac and skeletal muscle, endocrine secretory cells, neurons, glia and oocytes. Thus, calcium plays an important role in contractile, secretory and other functions throughout the body. Numerous neurotransmitters (e.g. calcitonin) and cations (e.g., mg^{+2}) can effect the entry of calcium into cells through VDCC's and CEB's inhibit Ca^{+2} flux through these channels. At present four major classes of CEB's exist (Table 7) and they act by decreasing Ca^{+2} channel opening. There is a

Table 7. CEB classification.

Class	Drug
Dihydropyridines	Nifedipine, nimodipine
Phenylalkylamines	Verapamil
Benzothiazepines	Diltiazem
Diphenylalkylamines	Flunarizine

tremendous heterogeneity of Ca^{+2} channels and different channel types may functionally predominate during different cellular electrophysiologic states (61,62).

The three CEB's currently used in the United States bind to different receptors associated with VDCC's. However, these receptors are functionally interdependent and binding of one drug to one receptor allosterically influences the others. Thus while verapamil, through an action on a distinct receptor will cause [^{3}H] nitrendipine (nifedipine type drug) to dissociate more rapidly from its receptor, diltiazem enhances [^{3}H] nitrendipine binding. These three CEB's do not directly block the VDCC but influence calcium conductance through the VDCC through receptors for which the endogenous ligands are not clear or discovered.

Given the complexity of interactions it is not surprising that different CEB's have predominantly different effects. Thus drugs of the nifedipine class are particularly effective in reducing the contractility of smooth muscle in blood vessels and have found use in treating angina and hypertension (63). Verapamil-type compounds are most effective where VDCC frequency of opening and closing is greatest (e.g., sinus and atrioventricular nodes) and are useful in supraventricular cardiac arrhythmias (64, 65). Diltiazem has overlapping effects and is useful for both angina and arrhythmias. VDCC's are ubiquitous in man and other possible therapies are just beginning to be explored. Potential uses include treatment of headache (66), therapeutic interventions designed to reduce cerebral vasospasm associated with subarachnoid hemorrhage (67) and irreversible cellular injury during stroke and cardiac arrest (68), as well as benefits for patients with esophogeal disorders, peripheral vascular disease, reflex sympathetic dystrophy, and myometrial hyperactivity.

CONCLUDING REMARKS

In summary, although pharmacologic antagonists form a heterogenous group of compounds, they have found a permanent place in anesthesia. The advent of a specific benzodiazepine antagonist will allow all four elements constituting balanced anesthesia--amnesia, analgesia, muscle relaxation and physiologic homeostasis to be managed in part with antagonist drugs, Fig 2.

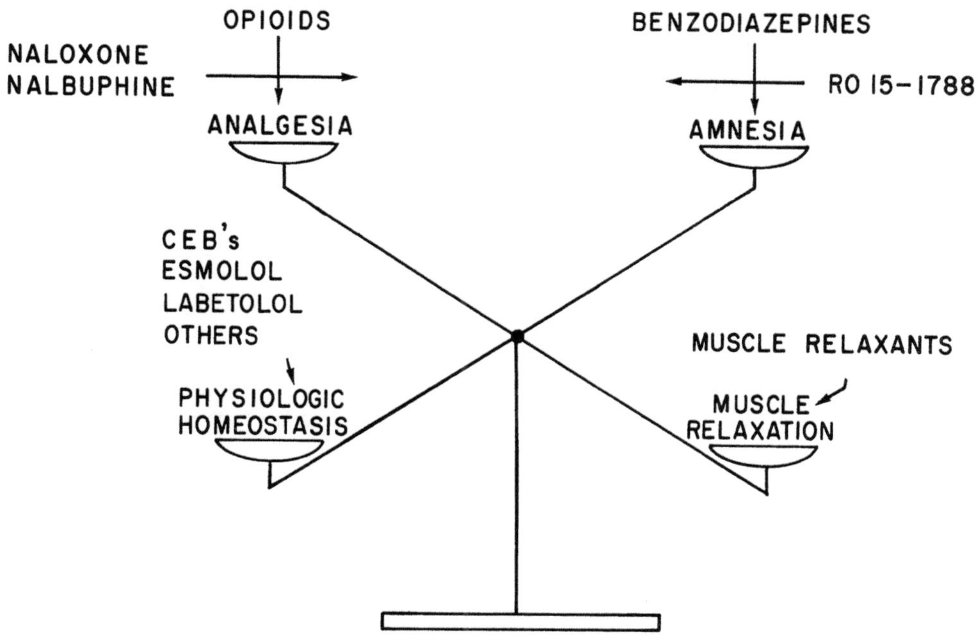

Fig. 2. Antagonists in balanced anesthesia.

Thus, pre-operative sedation or anesthetic induction with midazolam or other benzodiazepines can be reversed when no longer needed or advantageous. Opioid effects can be moderated if respiratory depression is excessive. Muscle relaxants help provide optimal surgical conditions and various other drugs, e.g., esmolol, help maintain physiologic homeostasis during stressful periods. As the biochemistry of cellular and organ systems is further defined and drug effects more specifically tied to molecular interactions, receptor functions and many more specific agonists and antagonists will be discovered and applied in clinical practice.

REFERENCES

1. Ahlquist, R.P. Am. J. Physiol. 153:586, 1948
2. Sheridan, D.J. J. Mol. Cell Cardiol. 18(Suppl 5):59, 1986
3. Flacke, J.W., Bloor, B.C., Flacke, W.E., et al. Anesthesiology 67:11, 1987
4. Braumwold, E., Muller J.E., Kloner, R.A., and Maroko P.R. Am. J. Med. 74:113, 1983
5. Slogoff S., Keats A., and Ott E. J.A.M.A. 240:1487, 1978
6. Kopova, C., Brown, A., Pappas G. Anesthesiology 48:28, 1978
7. Erhardt, P.W., Woo, C.M., Anderson, W.G., and Gorczynski, R.J. J. Med. Chem. 25:1408, 1982
8. Gorczynki, R.J. Am. J. Cardiol. 56:3F, 1985
9. Gray, R.J., Bateman, T.M., Czer, L.S.C., Conklin, C., Matlof, J.M. Am. J. Cardio. 56:49F, 1985
10. Richards, D.A. Br. J. Clin. Pharmacol. 3:721S, 1976
11. Carey, B. and Whalley, E.T. J. Pharm. Pharmacol. 31:791, 1979
12. Prichard, B.N.C., Boakes, A.J., Thompson, F.D., and Joekes, A.M. Clin. Sci. Molec. Med. 48:975, 1975
13. Carter, B.L. Drug Intelligence and Clinical Pharmacy 17:704, 1983
14. Wallin, J.D., and O'Neill, W.M., Jr. Arch. Int. Med. 143:485, 1983
15. Larsson, K. Eur. J. Respir. Dis. 63:221-230, 1982
16. Philbin, D.M., Mass J., Akins, C.W., et al. Anesthesiology 55:292, 1987
17. Mendelson, C.L. Am. J. Obstet. Gynecol. 52:191, 1946
18. Stoelting, R.K. Anesth. Analg. 57:675, 1978
19. Malinisk, K., and Vakil, A.H. Anesth. Analg. 58:309, 1979
20. Nathan, R.A., Segal, N., Glover, G.C., et al. Am. Rev. Respir. Dis. 120:1251, 1979

21. Mohler, H., and Okada, T. Science 198:849-881, 1977
22. Squires, R.F., and Braestrup, C. Nature 266:732, 1977
23. Hunkeler, W., Mohler, H., Pieri, L, et al. Nature 290:514, 1981
24. Darragh, A., Lambe, R., Kenny, M., and Brick I. Eur. J. Clin. Pharmacol. 24:569, 1983
25. Lauren, P.M., Schwilden, H., Streckel, H., and Greenblatt, D.J. Anesthesiology 63:61, 1985
26. Kirkegaard, L, Knudsen, L., Jensen, S., and Kruse A. Anaesthesia 41:1184, 1986
27. Abernathy, D.R., Arendt, R.M., Lauren, P.M., and Greenblatt, D.J. Pharmacology 26:285, 1983
28. Gordon G, Grundy E.M., Al-Khudhairi, D., Anderson, D.J., and Whitwam, J.G. Br. J. Anaesth. 56:1161, 1984
29. Klatz, U., Duka, T., Doraco, R., and Doenicke, A. Br. J. Clin. Pharmacol. 1:95, 1985
30. Turski L, Havemann, U, and Kuschinsky, K. Life Sci. 33(Sup I): 7-55, 1983
31. Roald, O.K., Steen, P.A., Milde, J.H., and Michenfelder, J.D. Acta Anaesthesiol. Scand. 30:341, 1986
32. Scollo-Lavizzari, G. Eur. Neurol. 22:7, 1983
33. Jensen, S., Kirkegaard, L., and Andersen, B.N. Acta Anaesth. Scand. 29(Suppl 80, no. 162):89, 1985
34. Sexton, J.D. Lancet Clin. 55:582, 1908
35. Eckenhoff, J.E., Elder, J.D., and King, B.D. Amer. J. Med. Sci. 223:191, 1952
36. Costa, P.J. and Bonnycastle, D.D. J. Pharmacol. Exp. Ther. 113: 310, 1955
37. Telford, J., and Keats, A.S. Anesthesiology 22:265, 1961
38. Azar, I., and Turndorf, H. Anesth. Analg. 58:524, 1979
39. Estilo, A.E., and Cottrell, J.E. Anesthesiology 54:352, 1981
40. Tanaka, GY. J.A.M.A. 228:25, 1974
41. Michaelis, L.L., Hickey, P.R., Clark, T.A., Dixon, W.M. Ann. Thoracic. Surg. 18:608, 1974
42. Flacke, J.W., Flacke, W.E., and Williams G.D. Anesthesiology 47: 376, 1977
43. Prough, D.C., Roy, R., Burmgarner, J., and Shannon, G. Anesthesiology 60:485, 1984
44. Partridge, B.L., and Ward, C.F. Anesthesiology 65:709, 1986
45. Taff, R.H. Anesthesiology 59:576, 1983

46. Andree, R.A. Anesth. Analg. 59:782, 1980
47. Latasch, L., Probst, S., and Dudziak, R. Anesth. Analg. 63:814, 1984
48. Tabatabai, M., Javadi, P. Tadjziechy, M., and Mazloomdoost, M. Anesthesiology 61:A475, 1984
49. Tran L, Durrani, Z, Barabas E, Wang XY, and Zsigmond, E.K. Anesthesiology 61:A476, 1984
50. Moldenhauer, C.C., Roach, G.W., Finlayson, D.C., Hug, C.C Jr., Kopel, M..E., Tobia, V., and Kelly, S. Anesthesiology 62:647, 1985
51. Blaise, G.A., McMichan, J.C., Nugent, M., and Hollier, L.H. Anesth. Analg. 65:S19, 1986
52. Zsigmond, E.K., Durrani, Z, Barabas, E., Wang, X.Y., and Tran, L. Anesth. Analg. 66:421, 1987
53. DesMarteau, J.D., and Cassot, A.L. Anesthesiology 65:237, 1986
54. Bailey, P.L, Clark, N.J., Pace, N.L., Isern, M., and Stanley, T.H. Anesth. Analg. 65:605, 1986
55. Bailey, P.L., Clark, N.J., Pace, N.L., et al. Anesth. Analg. 66: (in press), 1987
56. Bradley P.B., Engel, G., Feniuk, W, et al. Neuropharmacology 23:1487, 1984
57. Ketanserin: The first pure and selective $5\text{-}HT_2$ receptor blocking agent. Janssen Pharmaceutica Investigational New Durg Brochure, Sixth edition, March 1982.
58. Davies, J.A.H., Beswick, T., and Dickson, G. Anesth. Analg. 66: 575, 1987
59. Peroutka, S.T. Neuropharmacology 23:1487-1492, 1984
60. Greenberg, D.A. Annals of Neurology 21:317-322, 1987
61. Miller, R.J. Science 235:46, 1986
62. Snyder, S.H., and Reynolds, I.J. N.E.J.M. 313:995, 1985
63. Nayler, W.G., and Horowitz, D.R. Pharmacol. Ther. 20:203, 1983
64. Linden, T., and Brooker, G. J. Mol. Cell. Cardiol. 12:325, 1980
65. Henry, I.D. Am. J. Cardiol. 56:1047, 1980
66. Greenberg, D.A. Clin. Neuropharmacol. 9:311, 1986
67. Allen, G.S., Ahn, H.S., Preziosi, T.J., et al. N.E.J.M. 308:619, 1983
68. Steen, P.A., Gisvold, S.E., Milde, J.H., et al. Anesthesiology 62:406, 1985

METABOLISM AND ELIMINATION OF NEUROMUSCULAR BLOCKING DRUGS: (1) NEW OBSERVATIONS ON OLD DRUGS; (2) NEW PATTERNS IN NEW DRUGS

J. J. SAVARESE, M.D.

This subject has undergone quite a bit of evolution in the last several years, because the production of shorter-acting relaxants requires that additional possibilities for increased rates and routes of metabolism be incorporated into the molecules.

All older, long-acting nondepolarizing relaxants show similar pharmacodynamic and pharmacokinetic characteristics because their elimination pattern is the same: basically, they are excreted unchanged in the urine. Little or no metabolism occurs, and alternate pathways of elimination, if they occur at all, are minor.

To this basic background, additional processes have gradually been developed to allow liver metabolism or elimination, ester hydrolysis, Hofmann elimination, and plasma cholinesterase-catalyzed hydrolysis.

RENAL ELIMINATION

The high water solubility of all relaxants allows easy glomerular filtration. This physicochemical characteristic, however, discourages uptake and biotransformation by the cytochrome p-450 system in the liver, because this enzyme system requires lipophilic substrates. If no other route of metabolism or elimination exists, relaxants will be excreted in the urine. In a patient who is a homozygote for the atypical form of plasma cholinesterase, for example, succinylcholine is relatively slowly eliminated unchanged in the urine.

LIVER ELIMINATION

Both d-tubocurarine and alcuronium have minor pathways of excretion via the bile. No metabolism occurs.

LIVER METABOLISM

Both pancuronium and vecuronium undergo de-acetylation at position 3 in the steroid nucleus. This occurs about two to three times more readily in vecuronium. A large amount of vecuronium is taken up and stored in liver parenchyma.

The new agent mivacurium is hydrolyzed by rat microsomes in vitro and is taken up by dog and cat liver in vivo. Consequently, some degree of handling by human liver is possible, but not as yet proven.

HOFMANN ELIMINATION

This pH and temperature-dependent process is really a chemical degradation, and not a metabolic (biological) process. In vivo, pH changes of less than 1 unit are unimportant in terms of affecting the speed of the Hofmann. A temperature decrease of 5-6° C, however, will slow the reaction to about half its usual rate.

ESTER HYDROLYSIS

This nonspecific pathway in atracurium may have some importance in man. Metabolites which may result due to this process may undergo further breakdown by Hofmann elimination, so that the Hofmann is the ultimate mechanism.

In either case, however, atracurium is inactivated by the first metabolic/degradative step.

Since one of the breakdown products of atracurium during the Hofmann reaction is laudanosine, a CNS-active tertiary amine, there has been some discussion of whether enough of this substance may accumulate during atracurium use to cause CNS symptoms. This appears very unlikely during even prolonged clinical use. Clinical studies of the problem are still in progress, although most of the evidence thus far does not implicate atracurium.

PLASMA CHOLINESTERASE HYDROLYSIS

This well-studied enzyme system which actively destroys succinylcholine has been given another substrate, the new short-acting nondepolarizer mivacurium (BW B1090U). Hydrolysis of mivacurium proceeds in the same fashion as in the case of succinylcholine, at almost the same rate. The new drug is inactivated by the first step in hydrolysis.

There may be some hydrolysis in the liver as well. The breakdown products have no pharmacological activity in the CNS, neuromuscular, or autonomic nervous systems.

BW A938U (DOXACURIUM)
ARDUAN (PIPECURONIUM)

These new long-acting agents, though no doubt primarily renal-excreted with little or no metabolism, may show a minor biliary pathway of elimination. Studies are in progress.

Table 1. Metabolism and Elimination of Neuromuscular Blocking Drugs

Drug	Metabolism	Elimination
d-tubocurarine	none	kidney (major pathway) liver (minor pathway)
metocurine	none	kidney (only pathway)
gallamine	none	kidney (only pathway)
alcuronium	none	kidney (major pathway) liver (minor pathway)
pancuronium	liver (15%)	kidney (major pathway) liver (minor pathway) Both parent compound and metabolites are excreted in urine and bile.
vecuronium	liver (20 - 40%)	liver (major pathway) kidney (also a major pathway) Both parent compound and metabolites are excreted in bile and urine.
atracurium	Hofmann elimination	kidney (90% as metabolites) no liver elimination
	ester hydrolysis	The relative importance of this pathway in man is not clear. Metabolites which develop as a result of ester hydrolysis may still undergo further break-down by Hofmann elimination.
mivacurium (BW B1090U)	active plasma Che hydrolysis	kidney (as metabolites) Little or no excretion of parent compound occurs.
	? liver hydrolysis or oxidation	? liver - as metabolites
doxacurium (BW A938U)	little or none ? plasma Che hydrolysis	kidney (major pathway) ? liver (minor pathway)
pipecuronium (Arduan)	little or none	kidney (major pathway) ? liver (minor pathway)

Prognosis Following Acute Renal Failure

Alan S. Tonnesen, M.D.

Regardless of the etiology, when acute renal failure occurs in the perioperative setting, the prognosis for survival is poor. In addition, the prognosis appears not to have changed substantially since the advent of hemodialysis 35 years ago. This presentation will explore recent data regarding prognosis and its prediction in patients who have developed renal failure.

Abreo et al (1) reviewed records of 55 patients receiving hemodialysis from 1962 to 1969 and compared with 46 patients treated from 1979-1981. Patients with causes other than ATN were excluded and the cases were grouped as medical, surgical and obstetrical.

Baseline Data for 2 groups

Factor	1960's	1970's
Age	46.8	57.9
>60	36%	63%
Medical	18%	41%
Surgical	73%	57%
Obstetrical	9%	2%
Non-oliguric	9%	20%
Nephrotoxic	9%	50%
Sepsis	35%	50%
Hypotension	53%	46%

Prognosis of Acute Renal Failure

The more recent group was older and a significantly greater proportion were of medical cause, specifically related to malignancies and nephrotoxins . The important toxins included radiographic contrast media, and antibiotics. Among the surgical cases, gastrointestinal and vascular surgery were the most prevalent groups. The number of complicating factors such as hypotension and sepsis were greater in the more recent patients, suggesting that sicker patients were treated in the later time period.

Mortality Rates by Diagnostic Group

Group	1960's		1970's	
	n	%	n	%
Medical	10	80%	19	79%
Surgical	40	73%	26	65%
Obstetric	5	20%	1	100%
Overall	30	55%	33	72%

The increase in mortality was not quite statistically significant

Pre-Hemodialysis Characteristics

Factor	1960's	1970's
Delay (days)	7	12
creatinine (mg/dl)	12.1	8.5
BUN (mg/dl)	139	111
Duration (days) *	10	21

* in survivors

The authors concluded that mortality in ARF is increasing due to treatment of sicker and older patients.

In reviewing ARF, Cameron (2) noted an 85% mortality in postsurgical patients and a 50% mortality in medical patients. Infection is a common cause of death. Complications include GI bleeding, septicemia metabolic acidosis, neurologic abnormalities and are more common in oliguric cases. Reported non-oliguric case

Prognosis of Acute Renal Failure
mortality rates are 17 to 44%, vs. 50-87% for oliguric cases. Mortality differs according to etiology: nephrotoxins 36%; hypovolemia 64%; cardiogenic shock 77%. Mortality is higher if creatinine is > 3 mg/dl (64%) vs. lower creatinine values, (15%). Risk factors for death include respiratory failure, jaundice, cardiovascular complications, hypotension, hypercatabolism, oliguria, age, central nervous system depression, neoplastic disease., hemodialysis, and ICU treatment. Patients with ATN who survive have a 60% chance of return to normal renal function.

Asbach et al (3) reviewed 100 cases of ARF caused by hemorrhage, trauma, crush, hemolysis or sepsis. The majority had a daily BUN increment of over 60 mg/dl, with a mean of 98 mg/dl/day. Nutrition was supplied by a formula containing 40% carbohydrate plus 40 g of essential amino acids. As much as 20 g of amino acids is lost per 10 hours of hemodialysis. The majority died of their underlying illness after regaining renal function.

Outcome according to major diagnostic group	% Mortality
General Surgery	83.3
Cardiovascular surgery	91.3
Urology	60.0
Trauma	75.0
Other	72.7
Overall	78.0

Lazarus (4) believes that current patients are older and sicker and thus, explains the persistently high mortality rate of ARF. He feels that aggressive nutritional support is the most important determinant of survival and that ultrafiltration is a means to achieve that end. However, data conclusively supporting that position is not available.

Lien and Chan (5) retrospectively studied 58 patients with

ARF treated with hemodialysis and performed univariate and multivariate analysis of 26 factors potentially associated with mortality.

Risk factor for death	Univariate Significance	Multivariate Weight
Hypotension after 1 week	*	
Ventilator requirement after 1 week	*	
CNS depression after 1 week	*	* (1.72)
Malnutrition	*	
Jaundice	*	
Shorter duration of hospitalization	*	
Heart failure	*	
Use of parenteral nutrition	*	
Age	*	* (0.09)
GI bleeding		
Male sex		
Prior azotemia		
Prior COPD		
Prior cardiovascular complications		
Number of prior risk factors		
Surgical cause of ARF		
Longer duration of oliguria		
Serum creatinine > 5 mg/dl		
Longer duration of hemodialysis		
Number of dialyses		
Enteral nutrition		
Pancreatitis		
Sepsis		
Bacteremia		
Additional surgery		
Number of complications	*	
Inotropic drug support after 1 week		* (8.39)

Factors followed by an * were associated with an elevated mortality rate when considered alone. In the multivariate analysis, only 3 factors contributed independently to the assessment of risk of death and use of inotropic agents was the major factor.

Rasmussen et al (6) studied 23 factors in 148 patients treated 1977-1979. One half required dialysis. The overall mortality was 53% (78 patients died, including 9 who had recovered renal function at the time of death). The discriminant equation was -0.5194 plus the weights listed in the table, with no survivor with a score more than 0.21. On a subsequent test population, no survivor had a score greater than 0.46 and 28 of 31 with scores greater than 0.15 dying in hospital and 30 of 31 within 3 months. The factors listed with weights, but not an asterisk, represent factors included in the equation, even though it was not alone statistically significantly related to mortality in this study.

Risk Factor associated with death	Significance	Multivariate Weight
Pre-existing events		
Age		
Chronic hypertension		
Prior heart disease		.1371
COPD		
Neoplastic disease	*	.3957
Prior renal disease		.2117
Acute clinical settings		
Aortic aneurysm resection		
Open heart surgery		
General surgery		.2086
Trauma		.3170
Septicemia		
Pancreatitis		.3498
Acute respiratory illness		
Acute cardiac illness	*	.4248
CNS damage		.1977
Potential noxious events		
Duration of hypotension		
Excess aminoglycoside		
Pigmenturia		
Dehydration		
Complications of ARF		
Bleeding disorder		
Oliguria	*	.3746
Sepsis after ARF onset		
Respiratory failure	*	.1960

Gillum et al (7) paired 17 sets of patients with acute renal failure prospectively and treated with either an intensive or non-intensive dialysis regimen. All patients had creatinine of 3.0 or higher, urine Na > 50 mEq/l, Uosm < 400, U/P Creatinine ratio < 20. The intensive dialysis group was hemodialyzed to maintain BUN below 60 mg/dl and creatinine below 5.0 mg/dl, while the non-intensive group was maintained below 100 and 8 respectively. The overall complications were similar between the groups and mortality rate was not improved.

	Intensive		Non-intensive
Number	17		17
Pre-dialysis characteristics:			
Age (years)	56.5		56.5
Non-oliguric	6		4
Delay until HD	5 days		7 days
Outcome and complications:			
Number of HD	16		8
Duration of HD	23 days		22 days
Mortality	58.8%		47.1%
oliguric		71%	
non-oliguric		20%	
Septic	8		11
Hemorrhagic	4		10
Cardiovascular	6		6
ARDS	3		2
Bowel infarct	1		1
Hepatic failure	2		1
Seizures	0		1

HD = hemodialysis

These studies have value in counseling the patient, family and ethics committees and ultimately health care payors. However, they do not shed much light on the important clinical questions which may lead to improvements in outcome. Studies more likely to give important clues should carefully analyze the actual pathophysiologic sequence leading to the ultimate cause of death. Second, whenever possible, patients should be classified into groups based on the presumptive etiologies, not based on epidemiologic factors such as admission to medical vs. surgical service, sex or age. In fact, renal failure is more an indicator of a very ill patient than it is a cause of death. Very few patients die directly as a result of renal failure per se. That is, fluid overload, hyperkalemia, acidosis or uremic encephalopathy. Third, a better understanding of the etiology and prevention of acute renal failure should lead to a reduction of the complications of ARF and its therapy. These include risk of sepsis, GI bleeding,vascular and peritoneal access complications, impaired nutrition , complications of the hemodialysis and peritoneal dialysis procedures. Fourth, well designed clinical therapeutic trials of continuous A-V filtration vs. conventional hemodialysis, the importance of nutritional support, optimal modes of antibiotic therapy during ARF should provide useful information.

REFERENCES

1. Abreo K, Moorthy AV, Osborne M. Arch Intern Med 146:1338-1341, 1986
2. Cameron JS. Intensive Care Med 12:64-70, 1986
3. Asbach HW, Stoeckel H, Schuler HW, Conradi R, Wiedemann K, Mohring K, Rohl L. Acta Anaesth Scand 18:255-263, 1974
4. Lazarus JM. Intensive Care Med 12:61-63, 1986
5. Lien J, Chan V. Arch Intern Med 145:2067-2069, 1985
6. Rasmussen HH, Pitt EA, Ibels LS, McNeil DR. Arch Intern MEd 145:2015-2018, 1985
7. Gillum DM, Dixon BS, Yanover MJ, Kelleher SP, Shapiro MD, Benedetti RG, Dillingham MA, Paller MS, Goldberg JP, Tomford RC, Gordon JA, Conger JD. Clin Nephrol 25:249-255, 1986

PULMONARY EDEMA: IS YOUR FLUID MANAGEMENT BREATHTAKING?

P. BARASH

I. Physiologic Basis

A. Pulmonary Edema:

1. Classic Definition = extravascular water content of lung abnormally increased.

2. Current Definition = change in rate of fluid and protein flow through the interstitium of the lung.

B. Starling Forces

Key to a discussion of pulmonary edema is the Starling equation which describes fluid movement across capillary membranes. Starling hypothesized that the sum of capillary hydrostatic pressure (CHP) and the tissue oncotic pressure (TOP) was exactly balanced by the sum of the tissue hydrostatic pressure (THP) and the plamsma colloid oncotic pressure (PCOP). However, in the lung, unlike other capillary beds, the tissue hydrostatic pressure is negative. Thus, the PCOP is the only force which theoretically moves fluid into the capillary. Subsequently, it has been shown that the capillaries are permeable to various proteins, including albumin. The Starling equation has been modified to account for this observation by the addition of the reflectance coefficient.

Abnormalities in these parameters increase the risk of pulmonary edema. Due to the effectiveness of the lymphatic system and other "edema-safety factors" the extravascular water content of the lung can increase by 47% before any abnormalities in pulmonary function are observed.

II. Plasma colloid oncotic pressure (PCOP)

Chief among the Starling forces that effect fluid flow across the pulmonary capillary membrane is PCOP. PCOP can be defined as the pressure exerted by plasma colloids across a semi permeable membrane (capillary endothelial wall) which tends to attract fluid into the intravascular space. PCOP helps regulate the movement of fluid between the intravascular and pulmonary interstitial space. The normal range of PCOP = 22-25 mmHg. Albumin (MWT=69,000) is the prime, contributor to the PCOP. Other blood proteins contribute the remainder.

Protein Contribution to PCOP

	MWT	GM%	ONCOTIC PRESSURE	% OF PCOP
Albumin	69,000	4.0	18.4	68.0
Globulin	200,000	1.2	1.7	6.0
Fibrinogen	333,000	0.3	0.2	0.7
Other		1.5	6.7	25.3
TOTAL		7.0	27.0	100%

The differences between oncotic pressure and osmotic pressure are:

	Plasma Colloid Oncotic Pressure	Plasma Osmotic Pressure
Measurement	Oncotic	Osmotic
Instrument	Oncometer	Osmometer
Units	mmHg	mOsm
Components	Plasma proteins	Electrolytes
Physiologic Site	Capillary membrane	Cell membrane
	Intravascular	Intracellular

III. Fluid Therapy

A. Crystalloid
- Ringer's Lactate
- Normal saline
- Dextrose

B. Colloid
- Albumin
- Hetastarch
- Dextran
- Whole blood
- Mannitol
- Plasma protein

One gram of albumin osmotically attracts 18-20 cc of fluid. In clinical studies, plasma expansion is more rapid with albumin (or colloid) than crystalloids. If speed of restoration of intravascular volume is not critical, than crystalloid will suitably expand the intravascular space, but at a slower rate. On the basis of a decreased in PCOP and potential increase in pulmonary interstitial water (pulmonary edema) advocates of colloid therapy claim that respiratory impairment may result if large volumes of crystalloid are administered. However, numerous studies have shown that PCOP doesn't correlate well with intrapulmonary shunt, and when administered under controlled conditions, there is no difference in respiratory performance between a colloid and crystalloid groups of patients.

C. Albumin: guidelines for clinical use

1. Appropriate Use

   Shock, burns, ARDS, cardiopulmonary bypass

2. Occasional Use

   Acute liver failure, RBC suspension media, ascites, with surgery, acute nephrosis, renal dialysis.

3. Additional Data Required

   Detoxification

4. Unjustified Use

   Under nutrition, chronic nephrosis, chronic cirrhosis

IV. Etiology of Pulmonary Edema

A. Increased capillary hydrostatic pressure

1. Cardiogenic
   1. Left ventricular failure
   2. Valvular heart disease (MS)
2. Fluid overload
3. Narcotic reversal

B. Decrease plasma colloid oncotic pressure

1. Hypoalbuminemia (nutritional)
2. Overhydration

C. Increased interstitial pressure

1. Expansion of pneumothorax
2. Removal pleural diffusion

D. Altered permeability (noncardiac pulmonary edema)

1. Drug	2. Physiochemical	3. Miscellaneous
Antibiotics	Aspiration	Sepsis
Darvon	Oxygen toxicity	ARDS
Librium	Smoke inhalation	Transfusion reaction
Aspirin	Fat emboli	

E. Lymphatic insufficiency

1. Silicosis
2. Lymphangitic carcinoma
3. Chemical agents (Bleomycin)

F. Unknown etiology

Heroin	Eclampsia	Cardiopulmonary Bypass
Neurogenic	Cardioversion	High altitude
Pulmonary Embolism	Pulmonary parenchymal disease	

V. Pulmonary Edema and Emergence from Anesthesia

1. D/C positive pressure ventilation
2. Decreased cardiac output 2^0 venous return
3. Hypoventilation
   a. decreased $PaCO^2$
   b. increased $PaCO^2$
4. Airway obstruction
5. Increased BP

VI. Treatment Pulmonary Edema

A. General

1. Increase inspired oxygen concentration
2. Endotracheal suction
3. Positive end expiratory pressure (PEEP)
4. Diuretics
5. Digitalis
6. Bronchodilators
7. Morphine

B. Specific Treatment

1. Reduce Capillary Hydrostatic Pressure
   LV Function
   a. Preload = Diuretics, venodilators
   b. Afterload = Vasodilator
   c. Contractility = Inotrope
2. Reduce Capillary Permeability
   a. Treat underlying problem
   b. Pulmonary capillary wedge pressure
   c. Antihistamines, ?Steroids

3. Decreased plasma oncotic pressure

a. Albumin

General Reference:

1. Fishman AP, Renkin EM: Pulmonary Edema. American Physiologic Society, 1979, Baltimore: Williams & Wilkins, pp 261.

References;

1. Albert RK, Lakshminarayan S, Charan NB, Kirk W, Butler J: Extra-alveolar vessel contribution to hydrostatic pulmonary edema in situ dog lungs. J Appl Physiol:54:1010-1017, 1983.
2. Baraka A, Moghrabi R, Yazigi A: Unilateral pulmonary oedema/atelectasis in the lateral decubitus position. Anaesthesia, 42:171-174, 1987.
3. Barash P, Chen Y, Kitahata LM, and Kopriva C: The Hemodynamic Tracking System: A method of data management and guide for cardiovascular therapy. Anesth & Analg 59:169-174, 1980.
4. Barash, PG: Circulatory Strategies in Acute Respiratory Failure. Current Reviews in Respiratory Therapy 2:161-168, 1980.
5. Barin ES, Stevenson IF, Donnelly GL: Pulmonary oedema following acute upper airway obstruction. Anaesth Intens Care 14:54-57, 1986.
6. Brigham KL, Kariman K, Harris TR, Snapper JR, Bernard GR, Young SL: Correlation of oxygenation with vascular permeability-surface area but not with lung water in humans with acute respiratory failure and pulmonary edema. J Clin Invest 72:339-349, 1983.
7. Brigham KL, Kariman K, Harris TR, et al.: Correlation of oxygenation with vascular permeability-surface area but not with lung water in humans with acute respiratory failure and pulmonary edema. Am Soc Clin Invest 72:339-349,1983.
8. Brigham KL, Woolverton WC, Blake LH, Staub NC: Increased sheep lung vascular permeability caused by pseudomonas bacteremia. J Clin Invest 54:792-804, 1974.
9. Calvin JE, Driedger AA, Sibbald WJ: Positive end-expiratory pressure (PEEP) does not depress left ventricular function in patients with pulmonary edema. Am Rev Resp Dis 124:121-128, 1981.
10. Civetta JM: A new look at the Starling equation. Crit Care Med 7:84-91, 1977.
11. Cooper JD, Maeda M, Lowenstein E: Lung water accumulation with acute hemodilution. J Thorac Cardiovasc Surg 64:957-965, 1975.

12. Cooperman LH, Price HL: Pulmonary edema in the operative and postoperative period: A review of 40 cases. Ann Surg 172:883-891, 1980.

13. Dohi S: Postcardiopulmonary resuscitation pulmonary edema. Crit Care Med 11:434-437, 1983.

14. Ebert JP, Grimes B, Nieman KM, et al: Letter to the Editor Reply. Anesthesiology 64:299, 1986.

15. Flacke JW, Flacke WE, Williams GD: Acute pulmonary edema following naloxone reversal of high-dose morphine anesthesia. Anesthesiology 47:376-378, 1977.

16. Frank LP, Schreiber GC: Pulmonary edema following acute upper airway obstruction. Anesthesiology 65:106, 1986.

17. Gabel JC, Drake RE: Pulmonary capillary pressure and permeability. Crit Care Med 7:92-97, 1977.

18. Gutupalli KK: Acute pulmonary edema. Card Clin 2:183-200,1984.

19. Helbert C, Paskanik A, Bredenberg CE: Effective of positive end-expiratory pressure on lung water in pulmonary edema caused by increased membrane permeability. Ann Thor Surg 36:42-48, 1983.

20. Klancke KA, Assey ME, Kratz JM, Crawford FA: Postoperative pulmonary edema in postcoronary artery bypass graft patients. Chest 84:529-534, 1983.

21. Kopman EA, Ferguson TB: Interaction of right and left ventricular filling pressures at the termination of cardiopulmonary bypass. J Thorac Cardiovas Surg 89:706-708, 1985.

22. Krause LM, Langdale LA, Rice CL, Gould SA, Moss GS: Does interstitial pressure oppose lung water formation? J Surg Res 34:510-514, 1983.

23. Lee DS, Kobrine A: Neurogenic pulmonary edema associated with ruptured spinal cord arteriovenous malformation. Neurosurgery 12:691-693, 1983.

24. Lorch DG, Sahn SA: Post-extubation pulmonary edema following anesthesia induced by upper airway obstruction. Chest 90:802-805.

25. Lowe RJ, Moss GS, Jilek J, Levine HD: Crystalloid versus colloid in the etiology of pulmonary failure after trauma: a randomized trial in man. Crit Care Med 7:107-112, 1977.

26. Lydon JC: Furosemide may be detrimental in the treatment of pulmonary edema. (Letter to the Editor) Anesthesiology 64:298-299, 1986.

27. Maggart M, Stewart S: The mechanisms and management of noncardiogenic pulmonary edema following cardiopulmonary bypass. Ann Thorac Surg 43:231-236, 1987.

28. Matthay M: Resolution of pulmonary edema: Mechanisms of liquid, protein, and cellular clearance from the lung. Clin Chest Med 6:521-545, 1985.

29. Matthay MA,: Pathophysiology of Pulmonary Edema. Clin Chest Med 6:301-314, 1985.

30. Milne B, Spence D, Lynn RB, Sleeman D: Unilateral reexpansion pulmonary edema during emergence from general anesthesia. Anesthesiology 59:244-245, 1983.

31. Oswalt CE, Gate GA, Homstrom MG: Pulmonary edema as a complication of acute airway obstruction. JAMA 238:1833-1835, 1977.

32. Pare PD, Warriner B, Baile EM, Hogg JC: Redistribution of pulmonary extravascular water with positive end-expiratory pressure in canine pulmonary edema. Am Rev Resp Dis 127:590-593, 1983.

33. Pavlin DJ, Raghu G, Rogers TR, et al.: Reexpansion Hypotension: A complication of rapid evacuation of prolonged pneumothorax. Chest 89:70-74, 1986.

34. Pavlin DJ: Lun Reexpansion - For better or worse? Chest 89:2-3, 1986.

35. Peterson BT, Ross JC, Brigham KL: Effect of naloxone on the pulmonary vascular responses to anesthetized sheep. Am Rev Respir Dis 128:1024-1029, 1983.

36. Popovsky MA, Abel MD, Moore SB: Transfusion-related acute lung injury associated with passive transfer of antileukocyte antibodies. Am Rev Resp Dis 128:185-189, 1983.

37. Rafferty T, Ljungquist R, Firestone L, Curtis A, Raven C, Hui S, Barash P: The plasma colloid oncotic pressure - pulmonary artery occlusion pressure gradient - A poor predictor of pulmonary edema in surgical intensive care unit patients. Arch Surg 118:841-843, 1983.

38. Rao CC, McNiece WL, Krishna G: Acute pulmonary edema after removal of an esophageal foreign body in an infant. Crit Care Med 14:988-989, 1986.

39. Rasanen J: Conventional and high frequency controlled mechanical ventilation in patients with left ventricular dysfunction and pulmonary edema. Chest 91:225-229, 1987.

40. Sgouris JT, Rene A: Proceedings of the Workshop on Albumin. DHEW Publication No (NIH) 76-925, 1975.

41. Shoemaker WC, Hauser CJ: Critique of crystalloid verses colloid therapy in shock and shock lung. Crit Care Med 7:117-124, 1977.

42. Sivak ED, Richmond BJ, O'Donavan PB, Borkowski GP: Value of extravascular lung water measurement vs portable chest x-ray in the management of pulmonary edema. Crit Care Med 11:498-501, 1983.

43. Slutsky RA, Peck WW, Higgins CB: Pulmonary edema formation with myocardial infarction and left atrial hypertension: intravascular and extravascular pulmonary fluid volumes. Circulation 68:164-169, 1983.

44. Snapper JR, Brigham KL: Pulmonary Edema. Hosp Practice 87-101, 1986.

45. Sprung CL, Caralis PV, Marcial EH, et al.: The effects of high-dose corticosteroids in patients with septic shock: A prospective, controlled study. N Engl J Med 311:1137-1143, 1984.

46. Tranbaugh RF, Elings VB, Christensen JM, Lewis FR: Effect of inhalation injury on lung water accumulation. J Trauma 23:597-604, 1983.

47. Tranbaugh RF, Lewis FR: Mechanisms and etiologic factors of pulmonary edema. Surg Gynecol Obstet 158:193-206, 1984.

48. Tullis JL: Albumin. 2. Guidelines and Clinical Use. JAMA 237:460-463, 1977.

49. Tullis JL: Albumin. 1. Background and Use. JAMA 237:335-360, 1977.

50. Vandyke WH, Jr, Cure J, Chakko CS, Gheorghiade M: Pulmonary edema after pericardiocentesis for cardiac tamponade. N Engl J Med 309:595-596, 1983.

51. Virgilio RW, Smith DE, Zarins CK: Balanced electrolyte solutions: experimental and clinical studies. Crit Care Med 7:98-106, 1977.

52. Ward HN: Pulmonary infiltrates associates with leukoagglutinin transfusion reactions. Ann Intern Med 73:689-694, 1970.

53. Weil MH, Henning RJ, Puri VK: Colloid oncotic pressure: clinical significance. Crit Care Med 7:113-116, 1977.

CARDIOVASCULAR PHYSIOLOGY OF CONGENITAL HEART DISEASE

Alan Jay Schwartz, M.D., M.S.Ed.

Classification of Congenital Heart Disease

Congenital heart disease (CHD) is comprised of a vast array of anatomic variations producing specific alterations of physiology which are manifest in a limited number of clinical presentations. The number of anatomic combinations in CHD are so numerous that they defy memorization. A simple and logical classification of CHD can be based primarily upon pathophysiology. This type of classification attempts to distill the myriad of congenital heart lesions into categories from which the answers to several basic questions are provided.

1. Is there an abnormal pathway for blood flow (shunting) through an intracardiac, extracardiac, or combined defect?
2. Is there obstruction to and reduction of blood flow due to a supravalvular, subvalvular, or primary valvular abnormality?
3. What are the consequences of abnormal cardiovascular (CV) pressures or volume which result from shunting of or obstruction to blood flow?
4. What are the consequences on the pulmonary and systemic vasculatures, and pulmonary and systemic blood flows?

The pathophysiological classification separates the congenital heart lesions into three groups. In two of the groups the primary problem is shunting of blood through abnormal circulatory pathways. Alteration of pulmonary blood flow (PBF) is the major consequence of shunt lesions. PBF will either be increased, resulting in a volume and/or pressure overload to the pulmonary circulation (e.g., ventricular or atrial spetal defect, patent ductus arteriosus), or decreased, resulting in a relative inability to oxygenate blood (e.g., tetralogy of Fallot). Also included in these groups are complex congenital heart lesions in which there is a functional shunt (e.g., common ventricle, transposition of the great arteries, truncus arteriosus) which may or may not be associated with an anatomic obstruction to pulmonary and/or systemic blood flow. These more complex congenital heart malformations have the same effect of either ↑ or ↓ the effective PBF. A functional ↓ in PBF occurs, for example, when desaturated venous blood is shunted to the systemic circulation rather than to the pulmonary circulation because of the presence of a common mixing chamber such as a single ventricle.

There is no shunting of blood in the third group of congenital heart lesions (e.g., aortic or pulmonic stenosis, coarctation of the aorta). The primary problem in this group is obstruction to blood flow. The major consequences of obstruction to blood flow include the increased ventricular workload(s) necessary to overcome the obstruction(s) and the relatively reduced circulation distal to the obstruction(s).

Cyanosis or CHF are the two major clinical states which result from the abnormal anatomy. Cyanosis occurs most commonly in lesions where (1) PBF is ↓ or (2) mixing of systemic and pulmonary venous return occurs (e.g. transposition of the great arteries). CHF occurs most commonly in shunt lesions with ↑ PBF. Excessive pulmonary venous return to the left heart results in pulmonary vascular congestion. Less commonly, pulmonary venous congestion may occur when obstructive lesions or myocardial dysfunction impair forward cardiac output (CO).

Pathophysiology of Congenital Heart Disease - The "Plumbing" Principle

The pathophysiology of shunting of and/or obstruction to blood flow is explained by considering two fundamental principles of physics; Ohm's Law and the Hagen-Poiseuille relationship. While neither of these are used quantitatively, in a qualitative sense they are very helpful in describing blood flow.

When applied to CV physiology, Ohm's Law relates blood flow to the pressuring generating it and the resistance impeding it.

Ohm's Law (Cardiovascular Equivalent)

$$Q \propto \frac{P}{R}$$

where:

Q = Shunt blood flow R = Resistance(s) to blood flow

P = Pressure gradient(s)

The Hagen-Poiseuille relationship describes the laminar flow of a homogeneous fluid through a rigid tube of constant caliber and length. When applied to CV physiology it is "assumed" that blood is a homogeneous fluid and the blood vessels are relatively constant size conducting tubes.

Hagen-Poiseuille Relationship

$$Q = \frac{\Delta P \pi r^4}{8L\eta}$$

where:

Q = Blood flow

ΔP = Pressure drop in fluid as it flows through a vascular channel

r = Radius of the vascular conduit

L = Length of the vascular conduit

η = Viscosity of fluid (assumed to remain constant)

In this relationship, $\pi r^4/L$ represents the cross-sectional area of the vascular conduit over its length. This is a more specifically defined resistance factor than that used in Ohm's Law.

Combination and modification of Ohm's Law and the Hagen-Poiseuille relationship yields a versatile learning tool which can be used to understand the pathophysiology of CHD. The reaggregation of these expressions results in a CV "plumbing" principle (Figure 1) expressed as:

$$Q \propto \frac{P \times D^4}{R}$$

where:

Q = Blood flow (cardiac output and/or shunt flow)

P = Pressure gradient(s) (across valve(s), outflow tract(s), and/or intracardiac or extracardiac communication(s))

D = Diameter(s) (of valves, and/or intracardiac or extracardiac communication(s))

R = Resistance(s) (to blood flow (ventricular outflow tract(s), cross-sectional area(s) of a vascular bed(s), and/or length(s) of vascular channel(s))

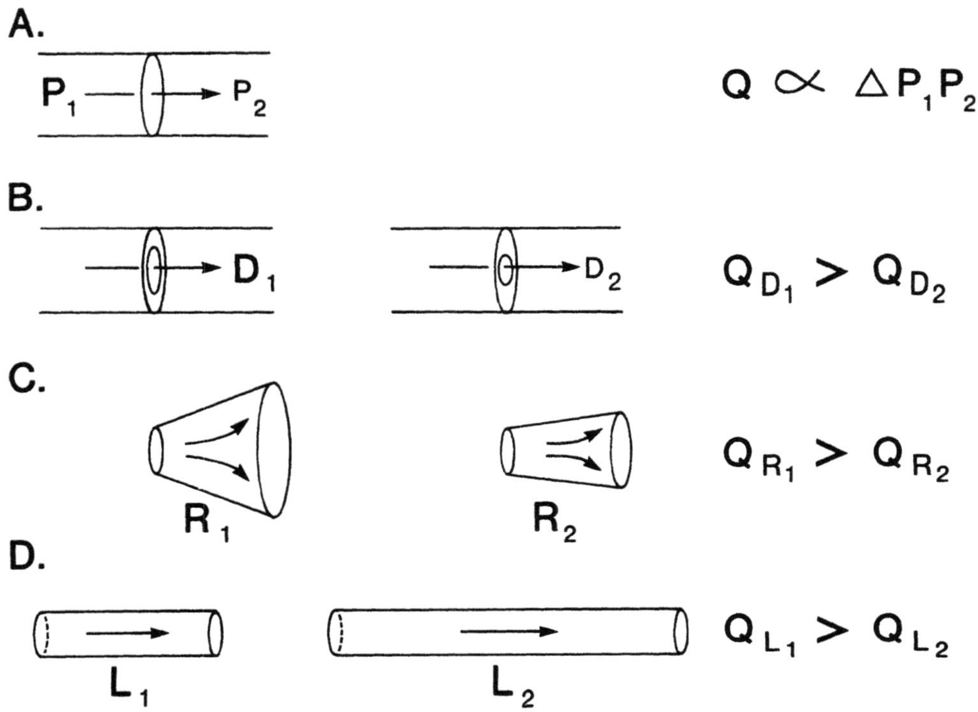

Figure 1: Schematic representation of the individual factors which influence the flow of blood through vascular channels. The quantity of flow is determined by pressure gradients in vascular channels, the diameter of the vascular channel, the resistance offered by the circuit into which the vascular channels empties, and the length of the vascular channel. Q=blood flow; Δ=difference between; P=pressure; D=diameter; R=resistance; L=length. A. Q is proportional to Δ P_1 and P_2. In the diagram, P_1 is > than P_2, therefore, Q is in the direction of P_2. B. Two vascular channels of different diameters are shown. Q through the channel with the larger diameter, D_1, is > Q through the channel with the smaller diameter, D_2. C. Two vascular channels of equal initial diamter (the opening of each on the left) are shown emptying into circuits offering different resistance. Q through the channel offering less resistance, R_1, is > Q through the channel offering more resistance, R_2. D. Two vascular channels of equal diameter and different length are shown. Q through the shorter channel, L_1, is > Q through the longer channel, L_2.

Applied Pathophysiology of Congenital Heart Disease

Ventricular septal defect (VSD) is an example of an ↑ PBF lesion (Figure 2). Blood is shunted into the lungs because left ventricular (LV) pressure is higher than right ventricular (RV) pressure, and right ventricular outflow tract (RVOT) resistance (including that contributed by the pulmonary vasculature) offers less impedance to flow than that of the systemic circulation. The existence of <u>any</u> shunted blood, and its total quantity is dependent upon the resistance to flow offered by the VSD itself. The larger the diameter of the VSD, the less resistance it offers, and the greater the flow across it from the higher pressure LV to the lower pressure RV and ultimately to the pulmonary circuit. This information can be conceptualized in the relationship:

$$\text{VSD } Q(\text{pulmonary shunt}) \propto \frac{P(LV>RV) \times D^4(VSD)}{R(PVR<SVR)}$$

where:

LV = left ventricle PVR = pulmonary vascular resistance

RV = right ventricle SVR = systemic vascular resistance

Tetralogy of Fallot (TOF) is an example of a ↓ PBF flow lesion (Figure 2). Blood is shunted away from the lungs because the muscular portion of the RVOT is obstructed (infundibular pulmonic stenosis) and offers more resistance to blood flow than the interventricular communication, i.e., the VSD, which is present. The VSD actually serves as a "pop off valve" that decompresses the RV which can not empty normally due to its obstructed outflow tract. The pressure in the RV, which commonly equals or exceeds the pressure in the LV, is elevated in response to the resistance of the normal pathway for RV emptying. As long as the SVR is relatively low in comparison to the resistance offered by the obstructed RVOT, the LV empties in a normal fasion and an additional quantity of blood will flow from the RV through the VSD to the LV and ultimately to the systemic circuit. This information can be conceptualized in the relationship:

$$\text{TOF } Q(\text{systemic shunt}) \propto \frac{P(RV>LV) \times D^4(VSD)}{R(RVOT>SVR)}$$

where:

RVOT = Right ventricular outflow tract

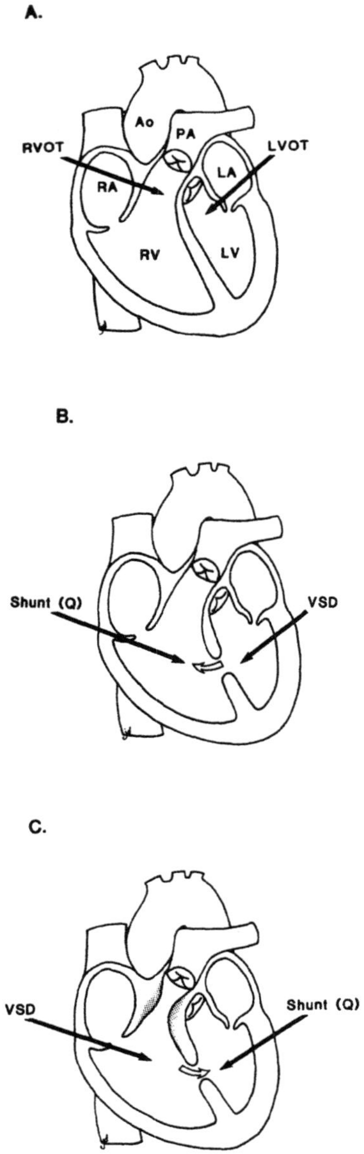

Figure 2: Diagrammatic representation of a normal heart and congenital heart lesions in which there is a pathophysiological alteration in PBF. Ao=aorta; LA=left atrium; LV=left ventricle; LVOT= left ventricular outflow tract; P=pressure; PA= pulmonary artery; Q=shunt blood flow; R=resistance to blood flow; RA=right atrium; RV=right ventricle; RVOT=right ventricular outflow tract; VSD= ventricular septal defect. A. A normal heart showing the anatomic relationships between the cardiac chambers and the outflow tracts of the ventricles. B. An ↑ PBF lesion is exemplified by a VSD. When 1) the VSD is large diameter offering low R, and 2) RVOT and PA offer low R, then 3) $P_{LV}>P_{RV}$, and Q, indicated by the open arrow, is left-to-right. C. A ↓ PBF lesion is exemplified by tetralogy of Fallot. When 1) the VSD is large diameter offering low R, 2) RVOT is obstructed (subpulmonic muscular hypertrophy indicated by the shaded areas), 3) RVOT R> LVOT R, then 4) $P_{RV} \geq P_{LV}$, and Q, indicated by the open arrow, is right-to-left.

Aortic stenosis (AS) is an example of a non-shunt obstructive lesion. The normal quantity of blood flows through the normal pathway. To satisfy the flow-pressure-resistance relationship, LV pressure must be markedly increased in order to overcome the resistance offered by the reduced diameter of the aortic orifice. This information can be conceptualized in the relationship:

$$\text{AS } Q(\text{systemic flow}) \; \alpha \; \frac{P(\text{LV}>\text{Aorta}) \times D^4(\text{Aortic valve})}{R(\text{LVOT})}$$

where:

LVOT = Left ventricular outflow tract

Anesthetic Application of the Pathophysiological Principles of CHD

Anesthetic manipulations alter the pathophysiological expression of CHD and have the potential to affect several components of the flow-pressure-resistance relationship. Cardiac depressant effects of anesthesia may limit the ability of each ventricle to produce flow (CO). If the ventricles' ability to generate pressure is affected, there may be a change in the pressure differential between chambers. Alteration in contractility may produce a desirable effect if an induced muscular relaxation unobstructs a ventricular outflow pathway which had been offering resistance to blood flow. Vascular effects of anesthetic manipulations may alter PVR and/or SVR. These changes may have direct effects upon the blood flow in their respective circuits which results from the interplay of a balance between the PVR and SVR. Specific examples will clarify these effects.

In children with lesions that ↑PBF, anesthetic manipulations are designed to reduce the shunt and increase systemic perfusion by increasing the ratio of right heart pressures to left heart pressures. While it is not clinically feasible to independently regulate the right and left heart filling pressures (preload), chamber compliance, or inotropic state, right and left heart pressures may be altered by manipulation of the impedance to outflow of the respective ventricles. Less blood may be shunted into the lungs by ↑ the ratio PVR/SVR. Increasing PVR promotes shunting of blood away from the lungs. Hypoxia, hypercarbia, acidosis, high mean airway pressure, sympathetic stimulation, and hypervolemia predispose to ↑ PVR. In the absence of clinically useful pulmonary vasoconstrictors, the avoidance of hypocarbia and the use of high mean airway pressures during ventilation (including positive end-expiratory pressure) may be used to maintain PVR. The use of vasodilators to reduce SVR, thereby increasing PVR/SVR, is of uncertain benefit. Vasodilators, including anesthetics, often exert similar actions on the pulmonary and systemic vasculatures resulting in no net change in PVR/SVR. Generalized vasoconstriction resulting from a high sympathetic tone due to light anesthesia, or from vasopressor administration, similarly may not alter the ratio of PBF to systemic blood flow.

In children with ↓PBF, anesthetic manipulations are designed to avoid further ↑ in right-to-left shunting. PBF may be promoted and right-to-left shunting ↓ by decreasing the ratio of right heart pressure to left heart pressure. This favorable alteration in the pressure gradient across the VSD may be accomplished by ameliorating the degree of right heart obstruction where possible, and by maintaining or elevating SVR. Manipulation of SVR in the presence of an elevated and relatively fixed impedance to right heart outflow will produce observable alterations in shunt flow. Increasing SVR generally promotes shunting of blood into the lungs. Light levels of anesthesia and the administration of α-adrenergic agonists predispose to maintenance or elevation of SVR. Infusion of phenylephrine into children with TOF produces ↓ in intracardiac shunting and ↑ in systemic O_2 tension. In this instance, the vasopressor ↑ SVR and impedance to left heart outflow relative to right heart outflow. This results in a decrease in the right-to-left interventricular pressure gradient that reduces RV to LV shunting. Decreasing SVR, on the other hand, promotes shunting of blood away from the lungs and could intensify the shunt and create cyanosis. Vasodilators and deep levels of anesthesia can predispose to ↓ SVR. If hypovolemia and systemic ↓ BP are superimposed on a congenital heart lesion with obstruction to PBF, both the right-to-left shunt and cyanosis are intensified. This physiologic sequence leads to shock and cardiac arrest if unreversed. Reduction in PVR may also help in promoting PBF. This is accomplished by hyperventilation with a high inspired O_2 concentration and avoiding high mean airway pressure.

The flow-pressure-resistance relationship can also be applied to the non-shunt obstructive lesions. Reducing ventricular function limits the heart's ability to generate a pressure gradient and produce CO in a setting in which obstruction to blood flow is present. The ability of the heart to eject stroke volume depends on the adequacy of ventricular filling and inotropic state. Excessive myocardial depression, hypovolemia, and loss of properly timed atrial systole are to be avoided. Adequate regulation of SVR is essential to provide important coronary perfusion pressure. Control of impedance to LV outflow is equally important, however, and excessive increases in this resistance to flow are to be avoided in non-shunt obstructive lesions.

Anesthetic depression of cardiac contractility is not always detrimental. In contrast to adults with valvular stenosis, AS and PS in children is often subvalvular (i.e., infundibular) in location. Forward blood flow and myocardial O_2 balance may be altered by modifying the degree of infundibular obstruction in these lesions. In TOF, for example, the RVOT is obstructed by a subvalvular muscular stenosis. Infundibular RVOT obstruction can be exacerbated by tachycardia and hypovolemia, which reduce ventricular size, and by excessive contractility. This can increase the degree of muscular contraction and obstruction intensifying the abnormal shunt. Systemic vasodilation may also impair RV infundibular outflow by causing a reflex increase in heart rate and contractility. Avoidance of excessive sympathetic tone, provision of adequate venous return, and control of SVR are desirable in this setting. The negative chronotropic and inotropic actions of anesthetics and β-adrenergic antagonists can be used to advantage to reduce an obstructing degree of muscular RVOT obstruction.

SUMMARY

Application of the flow-pressure-resistance relationship, i.e., the "plumbing" principle enables one to understand the pathophysiology of CHD and selection of an anesthetic technique for children with these lesions.

Suggested Reading

1. Fink BW: Congenital Heart Disease: A Deductive Approach to its Diagnosis, 2nd ed. Chicago: Year Book Medical, 1985
2. Kawabori I: Pediatr Clin North Am 25:759-795, 1978
3. Moore RA: Anesthesiol Rev 8(no. 12):23-29, 1981
4. Schwartz AJ, Campbell FW: In Pediatric Cardiac Anesthesia, Edited by C. Lake, Appleton-Century-Crofts, in press, 1987
5. Schwartz AJ, Jobes DR: Congenital heart disease-Special anesthetic considerations. In Cardiac Anesthesia, Conahan TJ (ed), Menlo Park, Addison-Wesley, 1982, pp 62-91
6. Stevenson JG: Pediatr Clin North Am 25:725-758, 1978
7. Young D: Int Anesthesiol Clin 18:5-26, 1980

ANESTHETIC MANAGEMENT OF THE CHILD WITH CONGENITAL HEART DISEASE FOR NONCARDIAC SURGERY

Alan Jay Schwartz, M.D., M.S.Ed.

INTRODUCTION

Anesthesia for the child with congenital heart disease (CHD) is fundamentally the same whether for cardiac or noncardiac surgery. The anesthetic plan is predicated upon an understanding of the cardiovascular (CV) pathophysiology and its clinical presentation (see Chapter: Cardiovascular Physiology of Congenital Heart Disease). The anesthetic implications follow logically from the knowledge of the alterations of physiology.

Perioperative Management of the Child with CHD for Noncardiac Surgery

A noncardiac operation for a child with CHD may be scheduled as an inpatient or outpatient procedure. A routine preoperative evaluation is supplemented by several specific considerations of the child with CHD. The child will often have undergone one or more cardiac surgical procedures in the past. It will be important to know the types of repairs performed (palliative or totally corrective) and how these impact the CV dynamics. The palliative creation of a Blalock-Taussig (BT) shunt, for example, increases blood flow to the lungs of a child with ↓ pulmonary blood flow (PBF) in pulmonary atresia. The total correction of tetralogy of Fallot (TOF) is associated with heart block and sudden death in a small but definite group of patients.

Associated noncardiac congenital anomalies are frequently present. Approximately 25% of all children with CHD additionally have a noncardiac congenital anomaly which often requires surgical repair. These are looked for and the presence of clinical syndrome complexes defined. The anesthetic plan may be further restricted by the presence of additional congenital malformations.

The parents of cyanotic children may report intermittent episodes when the child has ↑ cyanosis. This indicates that a reactive pulmonary vasoconstriction is superimposed upon an anatomically ↓ PBF intensifying the hypoxia. They may report that the child squats to alleviate this. Squatting ↑ systemic vascular resistance (SVR) and counterbalances shunting away from the lungs. Episodic reactive pulmonary vasoconstriction ("Tet spell") may occur in the perioperative period and is minimized by adequate sedation and minimal stimulation. β-adrenergic blocking agents employed to reduce right ventricular outflow tract (RVOT) obstruction and its associated cyanosis, will be continued up to the time of anesthetic induction.

When cyanosis is present there is an associated polycythemia to ↑ O_2 carrying capacity. The ↑ hematocrit may predispose the child to thrombotic complications. Perioperative fluid management will be designed to prevent further hemoconcentration. In addition, there is a thrombocytosis. Platelet function, however, is abnormal and clotting factors are often reduced resulting in coagulopathies.

Congestive heart failure (CHF) is quite common in CHD. CHF is a result of the increased cardiac work load associated with shunts or obstructive lesions. Maximal medical management of CHF is recommended prior to anesthesia.

The child found to have an undiagnosed heart murmur during preanesthetic evaluation deserves consultation by a cardiologist or experienced pediatrician in order to determine whether the murmur is suggestive of organic CHD or is functional. The risks of bacterial endocarditis (BE) and systemic air embolization in the presence of unrecognized cardiac defects mandate that even the asymptomatic child with a new murmur be evaluated prior to surgery.

Antibiotic prophylaxis against BE is indicated for children with CHD undergoing many noncardiac operations. Transient bactermia is common during "dirty" operations wherein the integrity of a mucosal surface is compromised. All patients who have undergone palliative or corrective cardiac surgery in the past require BE prophylaxis. The only exceptions are patent ductus arteriosus ligations and primary closure (without a patch) of a secundum atrial septal defect (ASD). In these two instances BE prophylaxis need only be provided for the first six months postoperatively.

The selection of preanesthetic medication is based on the child's age, psychological development, and CV function and is intended to alleviate psychological and CV stress prior to and during anesthetic induction. This will reduce the likelihood of excitement and sympathetic stimulation which may predispose to ↑ pulmonary vascular resistance (PVR), ↑ SVR, or ↑ RVOT or ↑ left ventricular outflow tract (LVOT) obstruction manifested as cyanosis or CHF. Children with compensated CHD may receive the routine institutional premedication by oral or parenteral route. Cyanotic children may be more heavily premedicated to reduce the risk of occurrence of a hypercyanotic episode. An anticholinergic alone, or combined with a reduced dose of sedative is appropriate for children with poorly compensated CV function.

The fundamental physiological deficits resulting from circulatory instability in CHD are reductions in systemic oxygenation and cardiac output (CO). Arterial O_2 saturation, heart rate (HR), and BP are parameters which reflect these hemodynamic events and each can be noninvasively quantitated. A basic monitoring setup, essential for children with CHD during noncardiac surgery, includes a stethoscope, ECG, noninvasive BP monitor, temperature probe, inspired O_2 concentration monitor, and continuous pulse oximeter for measurement of arterial O_2 saturation. End-tidal expired CO_2 measurement is increasingly used as a routine monitor. The site of BP measurement may be limited by previous cardiac surgery. A previous BT shunt, for example, prohibits use of the affected arm for accurate BP determination.

Establishment of intravenous access (IV) is a wise precaution for children with CHD no matter how minor the surgical procedure. This does introduce the problem of air bubbles. The introduction of air bubbles into the vasculature of the child with CHD who has shunting of blood may be disastrous. Bubbles in the venous blood may be shunted to the arterial circulation and result in an air embolus. Air embolus is possible even when the shunting is reported to be unfavorable to systemic embolization, i.e., ↑ PBF lesions.

The best safeguard against venous to arterial air or particulate embolus is meticulous prophylaxis. IV tubing, connection sites, stopcocks and injection ports must be free of air prior to connection to the child. Injection into an IV line is performed with care not to introduce air or particulate matter.

Full resuscitative capabilities must be available in the perioperative locations for care of children with CHD. Resuscitation drugs may be available or mixed up in appropriate concentrations ready for use. A defibrillator must be in close proximity.

Induction of Anesthesia - Uptake and Distribution of Anesthetic Agents in the Patient with CHD

There are no specifically indicated anesthetic techniques for specific CHD lesions. Whatever anesthetic technique and agents selected, the goal remains control of hemodynamic variables within the limits imposed by the CHD lesion and state of compensation of the child at the time of anesthesia and surgery.

The choice of anesthetic induction technique depends on the child's age and psychological preparedness, whether an IV line is present, the child's CV status, and the anticipated CV effects of the anesthetic agents. Anesthetic induction may be influenced by factors which alter the uptake and distribution of inhalation or IV agents in patients with CHD.

Alveolar concentration of anesthetic ultimately determines depth of anesthesia. Increasing inspired concentration and alveolar ventilation ↑ alveolar anesthetic. Decreasing CO, blood solubility and the alveolar to mixed venous anesthetic partial pressure difference ↑ alveolar anesthetic. The uptake and distribution of anesthetic in the child with CHD and shunting of blood is a result of the interplay of all of the factors which alter alveolar anesthetic level. The following exemplifies the interdependence of all of these factors on anesthetic induction.

Induction of inhalation anesthesia in a child with CHD and ↑ PBF:

Assumptions:

1. Constant inspired anesthetic partial pressure.
2. Rapid initial rise in alveolar partial pressure approximating inspired anesthetic partial pressure.
3. Tissue groups receive normal CO.
4. Shunt results in augmentation of PBF.
5. Full anesthetic equilibration between alveoli and pulmonary blood during first circulation through lungs.

Occurrences:

1. Shunt blood acquires no additional anesthetic during recirculation through lungs.

2. Systemic arterial blood delivers anesthetic to tissues depending upon regional CO, and blood and tissue solubilities.
3. Initially, the systemic venous blood is fully desaturated upon its return to the lungs where it fully equilibrates with the alveolar partial pressure of anesthetic.

Consequence:

1. A shunt which ↑ PBF does not affect uptake and distribution of inhalation anesthetics as long as alveolar partial pressure and systemic CO do not rise.

Under different conditions of inspired anesthetic concentration, alveolar ventilation, pulmonary and systemic COs, and tissue delivery and solubility, the effect of the shunt on uptake and distribution may be quite different from the above example. With ↓ PBF lesions, there is less blood contact with alveoli reducing blood anesthetic levels. In children with ↓ PBF of an amount sufficient to result in cyanosis, the limitation of blood-alveolar contact delays uptake and distribution.

Uptake and distribution of IV agents may also be affected by shunting of blood. This is recognized by examining CO curves from children with shunt blood flow.

In clinical practice, the effect of a shunt alteration in PBF can often be offset by the appropriate dose adjustment of administered inhalation or IV agents.

Choice of Anesthetic

Volatile anesthetic agents are widely used in the management of children with CHD. Halothane and enflurane, coupled with nitrous oxide, provide a smooth mask induction. Halothane, enflurane and isoflurane, permit the delivery of 100% O_2. The CV effects of the volatile agents are dose-related and titratable, and are well tolerated by most children with CHD. The hemodynamic actions of the drugs may be used to advantage in some children. The negative chronotropic and inotropic actions of halothane may reduce the degree of ventricular outflow obstruction and promote forward ventricular output. The potential hazards of volatile anesthetics are generally related to relative anesthetic overdose. Myocardial depression resulting from excessive dose may compromise CO and produce ↓ BP or diminish PBF and systemic oxygenation.

Nitrous Oxide (N_2O) is widely used to supplement volatile anesthetics. The use of N_2O following induction in cyanotic children with ↓ PBF lesions or mixing lesions is debated. In addition to the potential hazard of air bubble enlargement, the use of N_2O precludes the administration of high concentrations of O_2. In addition, N_2O has been shown to result in ↑ PVR in children with acyanotic CHD. The ↓ PBF and ↑ R→L shunting resulting from an elevated PVR/SVR ratio suggest that this agent be used cautiously, if at all, following induction in cyanotic children and those with pulmonary vascular disease.

High dose narcotic techniques are often used during surgical repair of CHD. Fentanyl (50-75 μg/kg) and O_2 administered with pancuronium to infants with an array of CHD produces only mild reductions in BP and HR. Prolonged postoperative ventilatory depression, however, makes high dose narcotic techniques impractical for most children undergoing noncardiac operations. The effects of smaller narcotic doses during surgical stimulation are not known. Low doses of narcotics may supplement a reduced volatile anesthetic dose or can be used in conjunction with relaxants and N_2O in a balanced IV technique. Light anesthetic techniques support cardiac contractility and maintain SVR. Balanced anesthetic techniques are well tolerated by most children with ↓ PBF lesions provided excessive sympathetic tone does not result in an ↑ PVR.

Ketamine is popular among many who care for children with CHD because of its hemodynamic actions and ease of administration. Intramuscular ketamine (4-8 mg/kg) may be used to induce anesthesia in an uncooperative child. Ketamine's sympathomimetic effect maintains contractility and SVR. IV doses of 2 mg/kg have not been associated with an ↑ PVR when studied in patients with CHD, including those with pulmonary vascular disease.

Thiopental (4-6 mg/kg IV) is a well tolerated induction agent in normovolemic children with compensated CHD. Reduced doses are indicated for those patients with compromised CV function.

Postoperative recovery of the child with CHD after a noncardiac operation is routine for the anesthesia administered and surgery performed. The intraoperative monitoring, venous access, and resuscitative capabilities are continued in the recovery area until discharge. Supplemental O_2 may be administered to the child with CHD during the recovery period. Ventilation is closely monitored to recognize and avoid hypoventilation and its detrimental CV consequences.

Summary

The child with CHD for noncardiac surgery does not present a major problem to the anesthesiologist. Anesthesia is planned around the anticipated surgical procedure. Understanding the pathophysiology of the cardiac lesion will indicate which anesthetic manipulations may alter CV dynamics. The pathophysiology will also clarify potential alterations in anesthetic uptake and distribution. There are specific perianesthetic protocols which are important when caring for the child with CHD for noncardiac surgery.

Suggested Reading

1. Campbell FW, Schwartz AJ: ASA Refresher Courses in Anesthesiology, Philadelphia, Lippincott, 14:75-98, 1986
2. Committee on Rheumatic Fever and Bacterial Endocarditis: Pediatrics 75:603-607, 1985
3. Moore RA: Anesthesiol Rev 8(No. 12):23-29, 1981
4. Morgan BC, ed: Pediatr Clin North Am 25:721-795, 1978
5. Rosenthal A: Pediatr Clin North Am 31:1229-1240, 1984
6. Warner JC, Fripp RR, Whiteman V: Surg Clin North Am 63:1003-1015, 1983

HORMONAL REGULATION OF RENAL FUNCTION DURING ANESTHESIA

Alan S. Tonnesen, M.D.

ANTIDIURETIC HORMONE

Physiology.

Production. Arginine vasopressin (AVP) is produced in the supra-optic and paraventricular nuclei of the hypothalamus and transported via axons to the posterior pituitary gland for storage. It is released from the posterior pituitary by neural depolarization.

Control of release. Release is stimulated by (1) hyper-osmolality (plasma osmolality > 283 mOsm/kg H2O) caused by solutes which do not freely cross the blood-brain barrier, producing levels of 0-15 pcg/ml; (2) by hypovolemia in the range of 8 to 15% producing levels of 10-100 pcg/ml; (3) by hypotension, which may produce levels of 500-800 pcg/ml; and (4) by a variety of other stressful stimuli such as pain, and nausea. Release is inhibited by hypo-osmolality and possibly hypervolemia. (1,2)

Actions. AVP causes constriction of smooth muscle including blood vessels and the GI tract; and causes an increase in permeability of the kidney's collecting ducts to water, thus allowing development of concentrated urine. The half life of released AVP is about 15 minutes. Levels between 0 and 6-12 pcg/ml produce the full range of urinary osmolality. Levels above 40 to 50 pcg/ml cause measurable vasoconstriction.

Effects of anesthesia and surgery.

Effects of Anesthesia on Renal Regulatory Hormones

Anesthetic agents per se, including narcotics, have little effect on vasopressin levels if hypotension is avoided. (3,4) Surgical or other noxious stimuli such as intubation cause elevations in AVP levels which are roughly proportional to the intensity of stimulation and, possibly, inversely proportional to the depth of anesthesia. Paradoxically, urinary osmolality appears to be less responsive to vasopressin in the anesthetized patient than in the awake state.

RENIN-ANGIOTENSIN

Physiology.

Production. Angiotensinogen is produced by the liver and circulates in plasma. Renin is an enzyme which cleaves angiotensinogen to angiotensin I, which is further degraded by angiotensin converting enzyme to angiotensin II. Renin is produced in the kidney and is normally the rate limiting step in angiotensin II generation. Angiotensin converting enzyme is found in capillaries and within renal tissue. Angiotensin II is the physiologically active product of the cascade. Levels are expressed in the quantity of angiotensin I released per unit of time.

Control of release. Renin release is caused (1) by loss of stretch of the renal afferent arterioles; (2) by beta adrenergic stimulation; and (3) by reduction in the rate of delivery of solute, probably chloride and/or sodium to the macula densa of the distal tubule. Hyperkalemia may potentiate renin release. Release is inhibited by angiotensin II, atriopeptin and possibly alpha adrenergic stimulation. (5,6)

Actions. Angiotensin II causes vasoconstriction; stimulates production and release of aldosterone; constricts the glomerulus, (7) thus reducing filtration area; potentiates nor-epinephrine release by sympathetic nerve stimulation; inhibits renin release; and stimulates thirst. The half life of Angiotensin II is 15-20 minutes.

Effects of anesthesia and surgery. (8-11)

Effects of Anesthesia on Renal Regulatory Hormones

Agents which cause sympathetic stimulation (e.g. ketamine) are associated with elevation of renin levels. If stimuli for sympathetic activation occur as a result of drug action or intra-operative events, renin levels will rise. Hypotension activates renal baroreceptor mediated release as well as catecholamine-mediated release. The dependence of blood pressure on angiotensin II levels during anesthesia is markedly inversely related to the patient's extracellular fluid volume and sodium balance.

ALDOSTERONE

Physiology.

Production. Aldosterone is produced and almost immediately released by the zona glomerulosa of the adrenal cortex. There is little storage, thus there is normally a delay of many minutes between application of an effective stimulus for release and elevation of levels, while new hormone is produced.

Control of release. Release is stimulated by hyperkalemia, angiotensin II; and ACTH. Hypokalemia and atriopeptin inhibit its release. (12,13)

Actions. Aldosterone causes a shift of potassium from the extracellular to the intracellular space; increases distal tubular sodium reabsorption by the kidney; causes structural changes in the distal tubule which ultimately result in potassium wasting.

Effects of anesthesia and surgery.

Anesthetic drugs appear to have relatively little effect (except for blockade of production by etomidate (14)) unless cardiovascular instability is produced.

ATRIOPEPTIN (ATRIAL NATRIURETIC HORMONE) (15-18)

Physiology.

Production. Atriopeptin is produced by and released from cardiac atrial myocytes .

Control of release. Release is inversely proportional to the degree of atrial stretch.

Effects of Anesthesia on Renal Regulatory Hormones

Actions. The overall actions of atriopeptin appear to be directed at causing a reduction in intravascular volume. Atriopeptin causes relaxation of vessels pre-constricted by alpha-adrenergic stimulation, but especially those pre-constricted by angiotensin II. There is little effect on unstimulated vasculature . Blood pressure is reduced as a result of a reduction in cardiac output. Peripheral venous pooling and a shift of fluid from the intravascular to extravascular space occurs. A major diuresis and natriuresis follow its release or administration, but there are weak if any tubular actions. The diuresis results largely from an increase in glomerular filtration rate which is caused by an increase in glomerular capillary pressure. The latter is related to a relative afferent arteriolar dilation and efferent constriction. The response of the total renal vascular resistance depends on the degree of pre-existing constriction, especially that produced by angiotensin II. Renin and aldosterone production are inhibited.

Effects of anesthesia and surgery.

The site of production and structure of this hormone has only been clarified over the last 5-6 years and its response to clinical anesthesia and surgery have not yet been examined in depth.

PARATHYROID HORMONE (19)

Physiology.

Production. The hormone is produced in the parathyroid glands.

Control of release. Release is inversely related to ionized calcium and magnesium levels.

Actions. Parthyroid hormone causes bone dissolution; stimulates intestinal calcium absorption; decreases urinary calcium loss; stimulates calcium and magnesium reabsorption by the distal nephron; increases vitamin D production; and reduces phosphate reabsorption by the proximal tubule. These actions elevate plasma ionized calcium.

Effects of Anesthesia on Renal Regulatory Hormones

Effects of anesthesia and surgery.

There is little information regarding the effects of anesthesia or surgery on parathyroid hormone release or actions despite the fact that hypocalcemia is a common finding in critically ill and anesthetized patients.

PROSTAGLANDINS (20-22)

Physiology.

Production. A variety of eicosanoids are produced by the kidney. As in other organs production and release are linked, with little storage. The prostaglandins may have local actions or may be carried to other parts of the kidney via either tubular fluid or blood. Thus, agents produced in the medulla may affect cortical events.

Control of release. The best characterized response of the prostaglandins is the protective vasodilator effect of the E and D series. When the renal vasculature is stimulated by vasoconstrictors, these prostaglandins are released.

Actions. The release of prostaglandins by vasoconstrictors blunts the reduction in renal blood flow. When this protective action is lost as a result of inhibition of cyclo-oxygenase by non-steroidal anti-inflammatory agents, excessive vasoconstriction may occur with a reduction in renal blood flow and filtration rate.

Effects of anesthesia and surgery.

There is limited information addressing the effects of anesthetics or surgery on renal prostaglandin production or actions.

REFERENCES

1. Robertson GL, Shelton RL, Athar S. Kidney Int 10:25-37, 1976
2. Dunn FK, Brennan TJ, Nelson AE. J Clin Invest 52:3212-3219, 1973
3. Philbin DM, Coggins CH. Anesthesiol 49:95-98, 1978
4. Lehtinin, Flyhrquist, Kivalo. Anesth Analg 63:25-30, 1984
5. Barajas L, et al. J Hypertension (Suppl 1):3-12, 1984
6. Briggs JP, et al. Renal Physiol 9:193-203, 1986
7. Ichikawa I, et al. Am J Med 76 (Suppl):43-49, 1984

8. Oyama T, Taniguchi K, Jin T, Satone T, Kodo T. Br J Anaesth 51:747-752, 1979
9. Brandt MR, Olgaard K, Kehlet H. Acta Anaesth Scand 23:267-272, 1979
10. Fray JCS, Siwek LG, Strull WM, et.al. Am J Physiol 231:1185-1190, 1976
11. Tanaka K, Pettinger WA. J Pharmacol Exper Ther 188:229-233, 1974
12. Field MJ, et al. Kidney Int 27:379-387, 1985
13. Marver D. Adv Exp Med Biol 196:153-171, 1986
14. Wagner RL, White PF, Kan PB, Rosentahl MH, Feldman D. New Engl J Med 310:1415-1421, 1984
15. Atlas SA, et al. Fed Proc 45:2115-2121, 1986
16. Laragh JH. J Hypertension 4 (Suppl 2):S143-S156, 1986
17. Needleman P, et al. New Engl J Med 314:828-834, 1986
18. Raine AEG, et al. New Engl J Med 315:533-537, 1986
19. Heitz C, Dulac H, Cuisinier-Gleizes P, Stoclet JC. Eur J Pharmacol 75:163-166, 1981
20. Makhoul RG, et al. J Surg Res 40:181-192, 1986
21. Raymond KH, et al. Am J Med (Suppl 1a):22-33, 1986
22. Gagnon JA, Felipe I, Nelson LD, et al. Am J Physiol 243:F265-F270, 1982

SAFETY AND EFFICACY WITH INTRAVENOUS REGIONAL ANESTHESIA

A.P. WINNIE

HISTORY:

The technique of intravenous regional anesthesia was first introduced by Bier in 1908 as a "new avenue to the nerves"[1]. The technique consists essentially of the injection of a local anesthetic into the venous system of an extremity which has been exsanguinated by compression and gravity and which has been isolated from the central circulation by means of a tourniquet. Bier's original technique was carried out as follows: The arm was elevated and an Esmarch rubber bandage was applied tightly from the fingertips to the mid upper arm to exsanguinate the extremity. A second Esmarch bandage was wrapped around the arm just above the exsanguinating bandage, as a tourniquet to isolate the circulation of the arm from the central circulation (Figure 1-A). Then the exsanguinating bandage was removed as far distally as the mid forearm, where a third Esmarch bandage was applied as a second tourniquet (Figure 1-B). Then the exsanguinating Esmarch was removed altogether. By this series of maneuvers, the upper extremity was divided into two compartments, the proximal compartment between the two

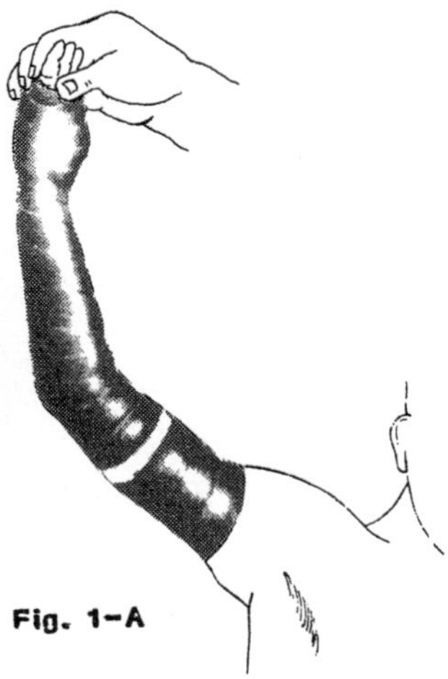

Fig. 1-A

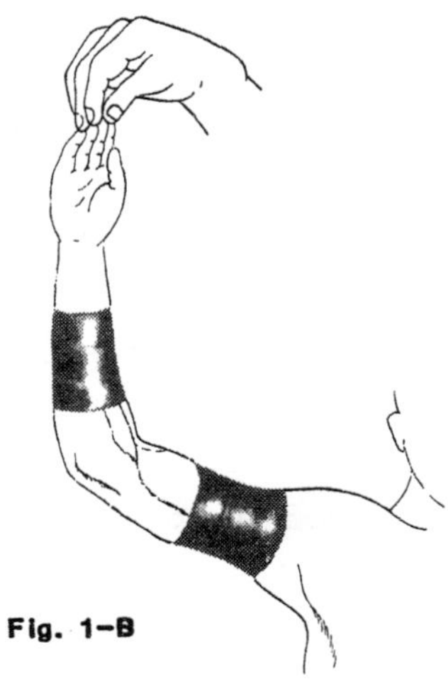

Fig. 1-B

tourniquets and the distal compartment distal to the more peripheral tourniquet. Bier then injected procaine, in his earlier report 0.25% and in his later report 0.5%[2,3,4] intravenously between the two tourniquets, usually in a distal direction in an attempt to overcome the valvular system of the veins and thus promote the filling of the entire venous system between the two tourniquets. Following the injection, Bier noted two types of anesthesia, an almost immediate onset of "direct" anesthesia between the two tourniquets and then after a delay of five to seven minutes, the onset of "indirect" anesthesia distal to the distal tourniquet. In an effort to delineate the mechanism of action underlying these two types of anesthesia, Bier carried out the same technique in cadavers, substituting methylene blue for the local anesthetic and then dissecting the tissues to determine the distribution of the injected dye. As a result of his studies, Bier concluded that the "direct" anesthesia which has an almost immediate onset between the two tourniquets is provided by that portion of the injected local anesthetic which immediately following the injection leaves the venous system to saturate the tissues, bathing the bare nerve endings. The more delayed "indirect" anesthesia distal to the distal tourniquet, he felt, results from that portion of the injected local anesthetic which does not leave the venous system but which is carried into the substance of the nerves via the vasa nervorum, where it produces a typical conduction block. Bier thus felt that his studies indicated that this technique, as he carried it out, above, actually provides a combination of peripheral infiltration and conduction block.

Bier pointed out that when this technique is utilized to provide anesthesia for extremity surgery, the patient might complain of tourniquet pain after a certain period of time, since the tourniquet isolating the entire extremity from the central circulation is above the anesthetized area. Bier offered two solutions to this problem, injection of a "bracelet" of local anesthetic simultaneously around the entire circumference of the arm just above the tourniquet or application of still another tourniquet immediately below the proximal tourniquet in the anesthetized area, so that the tourniquet producing the pain could be removed. Certainly, Bier was well ahead of his time in anticipating the "double tourniquet" technique utilized today.

Bier also stated that the tourniquet below the elbow could be omitted from the technique so that "direct anesthesia" could be provided throughout the entire area distal to the isolation tourniquet, which, of course, provided a much more rapid onset of anesthesia in the distal portion of the extremity. While Bier did not apparently utilize this variant of his original technique in any of his reported cases, description of this alternative technique is characteristic of the creative genius of the surgeon, to whom we are also indebted for the introduction of spinal anesthesia into clinical practice.

In spite of the fact that Bier reported the successful application of his technique in a multitude of surgical cases, reports by others of experience with this technique was not forthcoming, perhaps due to the fact that brachial plexus block by both the supraclavicular and the axillary routes was introduced only three years later, and was very rapidly adopted by many surgeon-anesthetists of that day. As a matter of fact, there is no further mention of the technique in the scientific literature until 1933, when Morrison(5) reported a large series of cases carried out with the alternative technique proposed by Bier, wherein the injection was made distal to a single tourniquet. Again, for many years following this single report, the literature contains nothing concerning intravenous regional anesthesia until 1946 when Herreros(6) reported a large series of cases carried out in his military practice. However, as with the report of Morrison, Herreros also failed to stimulate interest in the technique, as no articles concerning intravenous regional anesthesia appeared in the literature until 1963 when Holmes(7) re-introduced the technique into clinical practice. Following the publication of Holmes' article, the technique of intravenous regional anesthesia rapidly gained widespread popularity for the first time, interestingly enough, fifty-five years after it had originally been described by August Bier. Undoubtedly, the availability of better local anesthetic agents and better technical equipment contributed to the delayed success of this unique form of regional anesthesia.

CURRENT TECHNIQUES:

In order to provide optimal results, the following techniques are rigorously adhered to at the University of Illinois Medical Center: After placing a double pneumatic cuff high on the upper arm, an indwelling plastic cannula is inserted into a peripheral vein. The entire arm is then elevated, and a rubber Esmarch bandage is wound under the arm spirally from the hand to the distal cuff of the double tourniquet in order to accomplish exsanguination of the arm. At this point the axillary artery is digitally occluded, and then the proximal cuff of the double tourniquet is inflated to 50-100 mm above arterial pressure, and the Esmarch bandage is removed. Compression of the axillary vessels just before and during inflation of the pneumatic tourniquet is important, whereas the pressure rises in the tourniquet, venous outflow is stopped before arterial inflow ceases, and therefore, without occlusion of arterial inflow, exsanguination of the extremity may be incomplete. Following inflation of the proximal cuff and removal of the Esmarch bandage, 30-50 cc of 0.5% lidocaine is injected via the indwelling plastic cannula, the precise volume depending upon the size of the arm being anesthetized. If complete neuromuscular blockade is critical to the successful accomplishment of surgery, then 10 mg of gallamine is added to the local anesthetic. About 10 minutes after the onset of anesthesia, the distal cuff is inflated and the proximal cuff deflated, in order to minimize the possibility of the development of tourniquet pain.

If the patient has an extremely painful injury to the extremity, such as a fracture, manipulation of the arm and application of the Esmarch bandage is virtually impossible. In this situation exsanguination can be painlessly but effectively accomplished by using a zippered pneumatic splint: the upper extremity is placed on the open splint, after which the splint zipper is closed. The splint is then inflated to a pressure well above arterial pressure, after which time the distal cuff is inflated, the splint deflated and removed. Whereas the application of an Esmarch bandage to a painful fracture of the arm produces excessive pain, as the pressure is increased in a pneumatic splint, the fracture usually becomes more comfortable, and this, of course, improves the ability of the patient to cooperate, and hence the success of the anesthetic technique.

Just as careful attention to the technique of exsanguination is essential for the success of the technique using the intravenous regional technique of anesthesia, strict adherence to several irrevocable rules concerning the technique for terminating anesthesia will virtually guarantee the safety of this technique and prevent the even rare occurrence of serious complications. The first rule is that the cuff must never be deflated less than 30 minutes after the injection of the local anesthetic agent, even if the duration of surgery is considerably less than this time. The only case of cardiac arrest reported following deflation of the cuff occurred when the tourniquet was deflated only a short time after the injection of the local anesthetic (since the duration of the surgery was extremely short)[8]. The second rule is that regardless of when the tourniquet is deflated, the deflation procedure should be "cycled", as follows: the cuff is deflated and then immediately re-inflated, after which time the patient is observed and/or questioned carefully for the occurrence of symptoms such as tinnitus, lightheadedness, metallic taste in the mouth, etc., or even for the appearance of signs of stimulation of the central nervous system. If no such signs and symptoms appear after a minute, the cuff is delated again, and again re-inflated for a period of a minute or so, again to watch for the possible appearance of signs and symptoms of systemic toxicity. If none appear at this point, the tourniquet is deflated and removed. The safety of such a cycling regimen results from the fact that each time the tourniquet is deflated transiently, only a small part of the sequestered local anesthetic is allowed to enter the systemic circulation, minimizing the possibility of adverse effects due to a sudden, sustained increase in the level of local anesthetic. Clearly, in the central circulation, if the tourniquet is simply deflated (and not re-inflated), all of the unfixed local anesthetic agent in the extremity will enter the circulation at once, and will simply enhance the possibility of the appearance of adverse effects.

REFERENCES:

1. Bier, A. Arch. Klin. Chir. 86:1007-1016, 1908.
2. Bier, A. Muench. Med. Wschr. 56:589, 1909.
3. Bier, A. Berl. Klin. Wschr. 46:477-489, 1909.
4. Bier, A. Edinburgh Med. J. 5:103-123, 1910.
5. Morrison, J.T. Brit. J. Surg. 18:641-647, 1930-31.
6. Herreros, L.G. Anesthesiology 7:558-560, 1946.
7. Holmes, C. McK. Lancet 1:245-247, 1963.
8. Kennedy, B.R., Duthie, A.M., Parbrook, G.D. and Carr, T.L. Brit. Med. J. 1:954-957, 1965.

MANAGEMENT OF SIADH AND DIABETES INSIPIDUS

Diabetes Insipidus and the Syndrome of inappropriate antidiuretic hormone secretion (SIADH)

Alan S. Tonnesen, M.D.

SIADH

Etiology.

SIADH is seen in association with 5 categories of disease: intracranial disease, intrathoracic disease, endocrine abnormalities, malignancy, and drug side effects. (1) Four different patterns of arginine vasopressin (AVP) secretion have been described in patients who met the clinical criteria for the diagnosis. (2) In type A, there may be erratic changes in AVP which are unrelated to the osmolality. In type B, the threshold for AVP release may be lowered, but the response to changes in osmolality is retained. The "osmostat" seems to have been reset. In type C, the baseline level of AVP remained elevated, above the threshold, but when osmolality is increased, the AVP levels rose appropriately. In these cases, AVP release could not be completely suppressed. In type D, the AVP levels were normal and related to plasma osmolality in a normal fashion, but the urine remained inappropriately concentrated. Thus, despite meeting the clinical criteria, these hyponatremic cases were not due to elevated ADH levels.

Diagnosis.

The diagnosis of SIADH is always based on exclusion of the

presence of normal stimuli for AVP release. There must be hypo-osmolality of the extracellular fluid with hyponatremia; a urine osmolality greater than "appropriate" for plasma osmolality; excessive renal sodium loss; absence of edema forming states; normal extracellular and plasma volumes; normal renal, adrenal and thyroid function; and the absence of diuretic drug administration. In critically ill patients it is difficult, if not impossible, to assess whether the extracellular and plasma volumes are optimal. (3)

Theoretically, it is not necessary that the urinary osmolality exceed plasma, only that the urinary osmolality be higher than "appropriate." "Appropriate" actually refers to the osmolar and water balance per unit of time. For example, a patient with a plasma osmolality of 270 Mosm/kg H2O who needs to excrete 700 mOsm per day and consumes 2000 ml of water and loses 600 ml of water by non-renal routes, should excrete a urine with an osmolality of 500 mOsm/kg H2O. If the same patient consumes 4000 ml of H2O, the urine osmolality should be 206 mOsm/kg H2O. If the patient's urinary osmolality is 250 mOsm/kg H2O, then excess total body water will accumulate despite the fact that urine osmolality is less than plasma. From a practical clinical viewpoint, neither non-renal H2O losses nor the necessary osmolar excretion can be accurately measured. Thus, a urine osmolality higher than plasma is nearly always required to make the diagnosis of SIADH. The excessive urinary sodium loss is explained as follows. Excess H2O retention results in expansion of the extracellular fluid volume. Volume expansion suppresses aldosterone release and is associated with decreased proximal Na reabsorption. While specific information is not available, it may well be that the latter effect is secondary to release of atriopeptin.

Management.

The first diagnostic priority is to eliminate the factors which prevent making the diagnosis. Therapeutically, the most important factor is to assess the degree of hyponatremia and its effect on CNS function. When the sodium level is very low (< 125 mEq/L) or has dropped rapidly, then it is important to stop further depression and raise the level back to about 130 mEq/L. The same urgency applies if CNS symptoms are present. When it is urgent to elevate the sodium concentration, administration of 0.9% or higher concentrations of sodium chloride is necessary. If hypervolemia is suspected or supervenes during therapy, administration of a diuretic will allow more rapid correction. A careful assessment of hemodynamic status is required and fluid should be administered to correct hypovolemia. This step is critical because the accepted therapy for SIADH is fluid restriction. If hypovolemia is the cause of the hyponatremia, fluid restriction will magnify the problem, not correct it.

Most other therapeutic maneuvers are useful only in the chronic management of SIADH and are of variable effectiveness. These include lithium to block the effect of AVP on the collecting duct, demeclocycline to induce a nephrogenic diabetes insipidus, and phenytoin or narcotic antagonists to suppress AVP release. Specific AVP receptor blockers are being used in the laboratory and may someday find clinical application both for therapy and diagnosis.

DIABETES INSIPIDUS (DI)

Etiology.

The differential diagnosis of polyuria includes nephrogenic diabetes insipidus (AVP resistance), hypo-osmolality and expanded extracellular and intravascular volume (AVP suppression) and central diabetes insipidus (AVP deficiency). (1,4) AVP resistance is seen in hereditary nephrogenic diabetes insipidus, renal dysfunction due to primary renal disease or secondary to systemic disease and drug induced resistance to AVP action (e.g. lithium, fluoride toxicity). AVP suppression may be due to primary polydipsia or to iatrogenic fluid administration. AVP deficiency is encountered in association with hereditary deficits, and surgical or traumatic damage to the hypothalamus or pituitary.

Diabetes Insipidus and SIADH

Diagnosis.

The diagnosis is usually suggested by the presence of polyuria in a setting of CNS injury or disease. A common perioperative setting involves pituitary surgery. It is necessary to confirm that AVP release should be present before making the diagnosis of DI. In general, this requires demonstrating hyper-osmolality with hypernatremia, although obvious hypovolemia or hypotension would also be effective stimuli. Substances such as urea and glucose which cross the blood brain barrier readily may cause hyper-osmolality but not cause AVP release, thus, hyper-osmolality alone is not sufficient. Diabetes insipidus is relatively unique in that the urine osmolality is uniformly low (< 100 mOsm/kg H_2O), while nearly all other causes of polyuria result in urine which is iso-osmotic to plasma.

Management.

The first priority is to maintain intravascular volume at near normal levels. The second priority is to prevent severe hyper-osmolality. If the patient is alert, the mainstay of therapy is to have the patient drink freely as dictated by thirst. This requires leaving the patient unrestrained and with an unlimited supply of liquids of his own choosing. In severe DI, this will not suffice and the patient may become nauseated or vomit, thus limiting intake.

If the urine output is less than 150-200 ml/hour (2 ml/kg/hour), no other therapy is usually needed. If the patient is unable to tolerate oral intake, then hypotonic IV fluids should be administered at a rate equal to urine output. If the plasma Na concentration is above 145 mEq/L, no Na should be administered in the IV fluid. If a diuretic has been administered, the patient should be observed for signs of hypovolemia while awaiting a waning of its action prior to more specific therapy. When intravenous fluids have been used to replace urinary losses, the rate of glucose administration may have exceeded the capacity for glucose consumption, resulting in hyperglycemia and a super-imposed osmotic diuresis. The latter confuses the diagnosis and renders vasopressin therapy ineffective. In such circumstances, glucose administration must be reduced or stopped and insulin considered. Insulin should be given in small doses, if at all, and hourly blood glucose monitoring instituted because glucose levels often fall rapidly to the hypoglycemic range. A blood glucose level and urine glucose dipstick test should be obtained to rule out an osmotic diuresis.

After confirming hyperosmolality or hypovolemia, and a rate of volume loss which makes replacement therapy difficult, aqueous vasopressin, 5 units, should be administered subcutaneously or intramuscularly. In resistant cases it may be necessary to infuse vasopressin continuously, intravenously via an infusion pump. The dose and interval of vasopressin should be titrated to allow the urine output to recover to about 150-200 ml per hour prior to the next dose. After the urine output is under control, extra free water may be administered to correct severe hyper-osmolality. Chronic therapy is continued with intranasal DDAVP, with doses adjusted so that twice daily administration is necessary.

Other maneuvers have been used in management of DI with limited success. These include solute depletion, chlorpropamide, and prostaglandin inhibition. Solute depletion results in hypovolemia with a secondary fall in glomerular filtration rate and an increase in proximal tubular sodium reabsorption. These two effects reduce urine flow even in the absence of AVP. Chlorpropamide potentiates the action of AVP by increasing interstitial osmolality. Prostaglandins block the collecting duct response to AVP, thus, blocking prostaglandin synthesis will potentiate AVP action.

REFERENCES

1. Tonnesen AS. In: Askanazi J, Starker PM, Weissman C. Fluid and electrolyte management in critical care. Boston: Butterworths, 1986
2. Zerbe R, Stropes, et al. Annu Rev Med 31:315-327, 1980
3. Nelson PB, Seif SM, et al. J Neurosurg 55:938-941, 1981
4. Hsu T-H. Compr Ther 10:6-10, 1984

TECHNIQUES OF BRACHIAL PLEXUS BLOCK

A.P. WINNIE

The concept of continuous perineural and perivascular space surrounding the brachial plexus from roots to terminal nerves simplifies conduction anesthesia of the upper extremity and unites the several schools of brachial block into a single school - that of perivascular anesthesia. Thus, just as with peridural technics, the space may be entered at any level - axillary, subclavian, or interscalene - and the extent of anesthesia will depend on the volume of anesthetic and the level at which it is injected.

This concept has as its basis the fact that the brachial plexus is enveloped from the cervical vertebrae to the distal axilla by an extension of the prevertebral fascia. The prevertebral fascia splits first to invest the anterior and middle scalene muscles, forming between them an interscalene space into which the roots of the brachial (and cervical) plexus emerge from the grooved transverse processes of the cervical vetebrae. As the roots pass down through this space, they converge on the first rib to form the turnks and then divisions of the plexus, which together with the subclavian artery invaginate the scalene fascia to form a subclavian perivascular space. Passing beneath the clavicle, the divisions of the plexus split and recombine to become the cords of the plexus, and as the subclavian artery becomes the axillary, the fascia surrounding the neurovascular bundle becomes the axillary sheath, which continues into the axilla forming the axillary perivascular space.

The development of an exact technic depends not only on a knowledge of the anatomy of the brachial plexus but also on the ability to locate this anatomy using topographic landmarks. These landmarks, however, are not bony, as previously thought, but rather muscular and vascular. Hence the perivascular technics described above utilize mainly the sense of touch. If you can palpate the interscalene groove, the subclavian artery, and the axillary artery, you can master all of the perivascular technics of brachial plexus anesthesia. Which technic is used in any case will then be determined not by the experience or bias of the anesthetist but rather by the site of the surgery, the condition of the patient, and the level of anesthesia desired.

AXILLARY PERIVASCULAR TECHNIC:

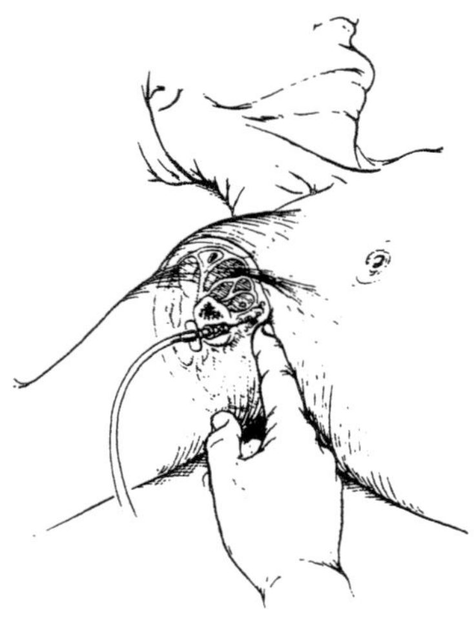

Axillary perivascular brachial plexus block (author's technique). A single injection is made superiorly tangential to the arterial pulse. The palpating finger collapses the vein and rolls it inferiorly, minimizing the possibility of venipuncture.

Our axillary perivascular technic is as follows: The patient is in the supine position with the arm abducted 90° and the forearm flexed and externally rotated so that the dorsum of the hand lies on the table next to the patient's head. The axillary artery is palpated and followed proximally as far as possible to the point where it disappears under the pectoralis major. At this point, with the index finger directly over the pulse, a 1½ inch 21-gauge needle is inserted just above the finger tip toward the apex of the axilla such that it will form a 10-20° angle with the artery as it is advanced. The artery is thus approached gradually until the definite "click" caused by the penetration of the axillary sheath is encountered. The tip of the needle now lies superiorly tangential to the arterial wall 1-1½ inches above the most proximal point of palpable pulsation. If properly placed, the needle will clearly pulsate. Following aspiration, 20-40 ml (depending on patient's size, sex and age and the level of anesthesia desired) of anesthetic is injected slowly with repeated aspiration for blood intermittently during the injection.

SUBCLAVIAN PERIVASCULAR TECHNIC:

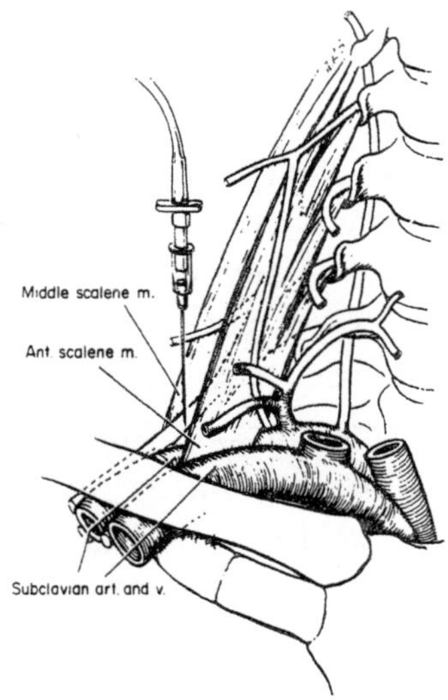

Frontal section of needle properly placed for subclavian perivascular block. Note direct caudad direction.

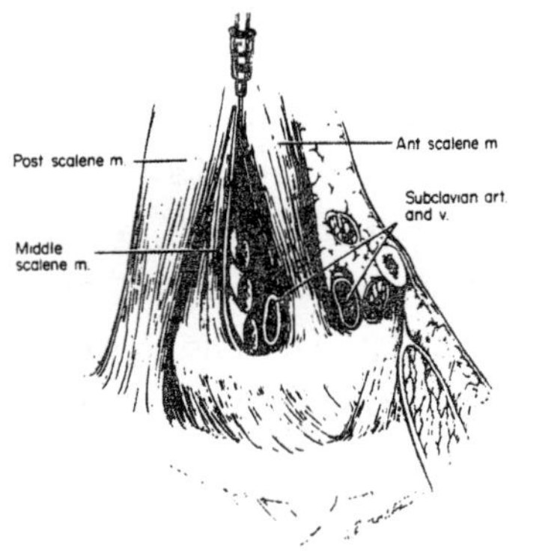

Sagittal section to show that the caudally directed needle lies in the longest axis of the subclavian perivascular space.

Applying the perivascular concept to the supraclavicular approach obviates the undesirable features of the classic technic, which is modified as follows: The patient is in the dorsal recumbent position with the head turned somewhat to the side opposite that to be injected. He is told to reach for his knee (to lower the clavicle) and then to relax the arm and shoulder completely. He is then asked to elevate his head slightly to bring the clavicular head of the sternocleidomastoid muscle into prominence. Beginning at the lateral border of this muscle, the index finger is rolled laterally across the belly of the anterior scalene muscle until the interscalene groove is palpated. The finger is moved inferiorly along the groove until the pulse of the subclavian artery is palpated as it emerges from between the scalene muscles. With the finger still on the artery, a 1½ inch 21-gauge needle is inserted above this point in a direction that is directly caudad but not mesiad but dorsad. The direction of insertion is such that the needle will be dorsally tangential to the subclavian artery in the longest dimension of the interscalene space, where the depth allows considerably more movement of the needle without its leaving the space. If the needle is advanced slowly the click of the needle penetrating the sheath may be perceived, though it is less pronounced than that of the axillary sheath; and a short distance beyond a single paresthesia to the hand confirms the fact that the needle is definitely in the perivascular space. At this point after the appropriate aspiration, the entire anesthetic injection is made. Usually, at the beginning of the injection, "pressure paresthesia", similar to that seen when anesthetic solution is injected rapidly into the caudal canal, offers further evidence that the needle is properly placed.

The direction of needle insertion, the use of a short needle, and the use of a single injection not only tend to improve the incidence of satisfactory results, but also to minimize the possibility of pneumothorax. Since the direction of needle insertion is parallel to the borders of the scalene muscles and since these muscles insert on the first rib, the position of the rib and vessel is located more precisely with this technic than with any other, although with this technic, in the vast majority of cases, paresthesias are obtained <u>before</u> the rib has been contacted.

INTERSCALENE TECHNIC:

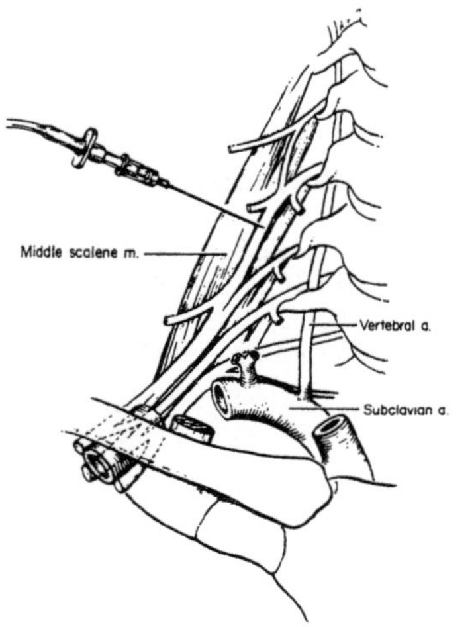

Frontal view showing needle properly placed for interscalene brachial plexus block. Note importance of slight caudad direction of needle (see text).

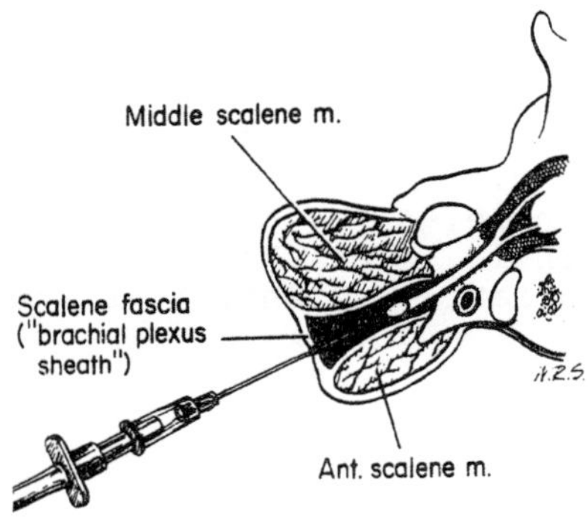

Cross-section view showing needle properly placed for interscalene brachial plexus block. Note slight dorsad direction of needle.

As pointed out earlier, as the roots of the brachial and cervical plexuses emerge from their grooved transverse processes, they enter the interscalene space formed by the fascia covering the anterior and middle scalene muscles. Since the majority of this space is above both the subclavian artery and the cupola of the lung, it would seem to be almost an ideal point to perform a brachial block at least from the point of view of safety.

The technic, as we have employed it, is as follows: The patient is in a position similar to that used in the subclavian perivascular technic. The interscalene groove is palpated, and the level of the sixth cervical vertebrae is determined by extending a line from the cricoid cartilage to the interscalene groove, and at this point, a 1½ inch, 22-gauge needle is inserted into the groove perpendicular to the skin in _all_ planes. The direction of injection is thus slightly caudad and dorsad as well as mesiad. The needle is advanced until a paresthesia is elicited and/or the transverse process is encountered. Once a paresthesia has been evoked the desired volume of anesthetic is injected.

REFERENCES:

1. Winnie, A.P. and Collins, V.J. Anesthesiology _25_:353-363, 1964.
2. Winnie, A.P. Anesth. & Analg. _49_:455-466, 1970.
3. Winnie, A.P. Anesthesiology _31_:577-578, 1969.
4. Winnie, A.P., Radonjic, R., Akkineni, S.R. and Durrani, Z. Anesth. & Analg. _58_:225-234, 1979.

LOCAL ANESTHETIC ADJUVANTS FOR BRACHIAL PLEXUS ANESTHESIA

A.P. WINNIE

Anesthesiologists are very fortunate today to have available to them a wide spectrum of local anesthetic agents, the duration of action of which ranges from about 30 minutes to twelve or fourteen hours or more. As a result, for a diagnostic, differential brachial plexus block on an outpatient in the Pain Clinic, 2% 2-chloroprocaine is utilized because it produces an intense block that allows the anesthesiologist to evaluate the response of the patient's pain to such a block; and then the anesthesia produced disappears quickly, so that the patient can go home. On the other hand, for prolonged surgery, such as re-implantation of digits, 0.5% bupivacaine is selected because it provides prolonged anesthesia, analgesia, and sympathetic blockade that extends well into the postoperative period; and while the <u>average</u> duration of surgical anesthesia is twelve to fourteen hours, there is wide variation in the duration, as evidenced by the fact that in some patients surgical anesthesia has persisted as long as forty-eight hours after a brachial block with bupivacaine. Furthermore, having selected a particular agent, in any given case the duration of anesthesia can be more precisely tailored to the duration of the surgical procedure by the addition or omission of epinephrine.

Certainly the greatest impetus to the utilization of brachial plexus anesthesia was the advent of the protein-binding local anesthetics, bupivacaine and etidocaine, since these agents produce anesthesia having a duration almost three times the duration they produce when injected into the epidural space; so they obviously provide the greatest benefit in terms of duration when utilized for peripheral blocks. Etidocaine is truly unique among local anesthetics in that it provides an extremely short onset of action and a prolonged duration, but it has not been a popular choice for brachial plexus block because of its tendency to produce a motor block that outlasts the sensory block by many, many hours. But certainly bupivacaine, and even tetracaine, have become increasingly popular choices for producing long-lasting brachial plexus anesthesia. The problem with these long-acting local anesthetic agents is that the time required for the onset of surgical anesthesia frequently causes an unacceptable delay in the surgical schedule. As a result since the beginning of this century there has been a continuing search for adjuvants and techniques which will reduce the onset time and/or enhance the block produced.

In 1885, just one year after the discovery of the local anesthetic activity of cocaine by Koller, Corning, a New York neurologist, demonstrated the fact that simple arrest of the circulation in an anesthetized extremity by compression or constriction proximal to the point of injection intensified the anesthesia, decreased the toxicity, and prolonged the anesthetic effect indefinitely[1]. For this purpose Corning utilized the Esmarch bandage, introduced just ten years earlier for the purpose of producing a bloodless field; and he pointed out that the method was readily applicable to surgery on all of the extremities. The use of such a tourniquet to prolong the local anesthetic effect of cocaine by arresting the circulation in the anesthetized area was widespread until 1903, when Braun introduced the use of epinephrine as a "chemical tourniquet" which rendered the elastic tourniquet unnecessary[2].

The use of epinephrine to prolong local anesthetic activity and to reduce toxicity was certainly a major step forward and remains today as, perhaps, the single most important adjuvant utilized with local anesthetic agents. However, several important points must be remembered concerning the activity of epinephrine added to local anesthetic agents:

First of all, the degree to which epinephrine prolongs anesthesia varies tremendously from local anesthetic to local anesthetic: for example, the addition of epinephrine to lidocaine solutions produces a 200% increase in the duration of sensory analgesia, whereas the addition of a vasoconstrictor to agents such as mepivacaine, bupivaciane and etidocaine produces only a 20 to 50% prolongation of anesthetic action[3]. Secondly, the impact of epinephrine on the duration of anesthesia produced by any given agent may vary, depending on where it is injected: for example, while the addition of epinephrine has little effect on the duration (and on the peak blood levels) of bupivacaine and etidocaine when they are injected into the epidural space[4-7], it has a much greater effect when these agents are utilized for brachial plexus anesthesia[8]. And finally, the effectiveness of epinephrine in reducing the rate of absorption of a local anesthetic and increasing the duration of a brachial block increases progressively as the concentration of epinephrine increases up to a concentration of 1:200,000, above which an increased concentration has no more effect on absorption and duration, but begins to produce significant, undesirable cardiovascular responses[9]. Therefore, except in the subarachnoid space, a concentration of 1:200,000 should never be exceeded.

In the late 40's and early 50's hyaluronidase became available and was utilized to enhance the spread and absorption of many solutions and medications injected into the body tissues. An early study indicated that incorporating hyaluronidase into a local anesthetic solution increased the normal area of skin analgesia resulting from an intradermal injection of local anesthetic by 40%[10], implying that the addition of hyaluronidase to local anesthetic solutions, by facilitating the spread of the solution, should reduce onset time and actually increase the incidence of satisfactory block. And, indeed, when Moore compared brachial plexus anesthesia produced by tetracaine 0.25% with and without hyaluronidase, he found that the onset of surgical anesthesia was reduced from 10-45 minutes to 8-15 minutes by the addition of hyaluronidase, while the success rate was unchanged[11]. As would be expected, the duration of anesthesia was also reduced from 4½-6 hours to 3/4th-2½ hours if epinephrine was not also added to the solution; but if it was, then the duration was unchanged by the hyaluronidase. Moore concluded that while hyaluronidase does markedly shorten the onset time of a local anesthetic, since it does not increase the success rate and since it does increase the incidence of systemic toxic reactions, the use of this adjuvant did not provide a significant advantage. In addition, since hyaluronidase is a protein, it can cause an allergic type of reaction; and in fact, three of the sixteen toxic reactions in Moore's series of 1520 cases were allergic types of reactions.

Potassium salts were first used as adjuvants to local anesthetics as long ago as 1912[12]. Theoretically, high concentrations of external potassium should reduce membrane potential, reduce potassium efflux from the cell, delay repolarization, and thus prolong the blockade produced by a local anesthetic. Bromage and Burfoot in 1966 used potassium chloride 120 m.mol. per liter in conjunction with 2% lidocaine in clinical extradural anesthesia and demonstrated a reduced onset time, an enhanced block, and a prolonged duration, but because an occasional subarachnoid injection of potassium produced convulsions and muscle cramps, these authors did not recommend its further use for epidural anesthesia[13]. Similarly, Aldrete and his colleagues in 1969 demonstrated that the inclusion of potassium chloride 180 m.mol. per liter doubled the duration of an ulnar nerve block using a 2% lidocaine solution, without any increase in local or systemic toxicity[14]. More recently, Kirscha and his co-workers demonstrated in animals that even the presence of a <u>physiological</u> concentration of potassium doubled the duration of blockade produced by a solution of lidocaine[15], thus obviating the risk of convulsions upon intrathecal injection or cardiac arrhythmia upon intravascular injection, but further work with this adjuvant has not been forthcoming.

In the early 1960's Loder reported that the addition of dextran to a local anesthetic increased the duration of block that resulted from it[16-18], and shortly thereafter this finding was confirmed by other investigators[19-22]. In 1967, Chinn and Wirojoatmadja[19] speculated that the dextran reversibly binds local anesthetics, forming a macromolecular complex that impedes uptake and distribution of the mixture from the injection site and consequently increases the duration of block. Rosenblatt recently tested this hypothesis by performing dynamic dialysis to quantitate the affinity for dextran and bupivacaine[23], but were unable to detect any binding of the two drugs. Furthermore, several recent studies failed to find any potentiation of local anesthetic duration by dextran[24-26]. Puzzled by these desparate clinical results and the failure of Chinn's theory of binding, Rosenblatt undertook studies that demonstrated rather clearly that the effect of dextran, and for that matter the effect of almost any agent utilized as a local anesthetic adjuvant, was simply due to the fact that the addition of dextran increased the pH of the local anesthetic, resulting in higher intraneuronal concentrations and hence enhanced local anesthetic activity[23]. As a matter of fact, they demonstrated rather clearly the fact that any adjuvant, urea, mannitol, or folate, would similarly enchance local anesthetic activity as long as the pH of the adjuvant was such that it would alkalinize the local anesthetic solution. This finding also explains the different results obtained by different investigators utilizing dextran as a local anesthetic adjuvant, since different commercial preparations of dextran have different pH's.

While these three approaches to local anesthetic potentiation have failed to gain clinical acceptance, and perhaps rightly so, there are currently three approaches to this clinical problem that have real promise: (1) compounding of local anesthetics; (2) utilization of the carbonate salts of local anesthetics; and (3) alkalinization of local anesthetics.

Let us look first at the compounding of local anesthetic agents: In general the short-acting local anethetics have a relatively rapid onset of action but inadequate duration for many procedures, while the long-acting local anesthetics provide adequate duration for most procedures, but have an unacceptably slow onset (with the exception of etidocaine). Thus, a logical solution to this problem would seem to be to compound or mix a long-acting and short-acting local anesthetic in order to take advantage of the rapid onset, spread, and penetration of one agent and the prolonged duration of action of the other. As long ago as 1949 Crawford and Chester combined procaine with tetracaine to reduce the unsatisfactory slow onset of the latter agent for caudal anesthesia for obstetrical use[27]. Subsequently, Moore[28], Bonica[29], and Lund[30] all evaluated the compounding of either dibucaine or tetracaine with chloroprocaine, hexylcaine, lidocaine, mepivacaine, or procaine; and it was Moore's studies based upon 474 brachial blocks carried out with the combination of mepivacaine and tetracaine with 1:200,000 epinephrine, that indicated this to be the most clinically useful combination evaluated[31]: this combination resulted in an onset of anesthesia in 5-8 minutes, complete surgical anesthesia in 12-25 minutes, and a duration of anesthesia that extended 4-5½ hours without any complications whatsoever in their series. Since 1972 at the University of Illinois Hospital we have utilized this combination, which the residents have termed "supercaine", in several thousands of cases and we have found that the onset of anesthesia is almost immediate, surgical anesthesia is complete from 10-15 minutes, and the duration of anesthesia extends to an average of 5-7 hours[32]. The slight improvement in onset and duration in our series of cases as compared with Moore's is probably due to the fact that we utilize a single injection into the so-called "brachial plexus sheath", whereas in the majority of his blocks, Moore utilized multiple injection techniques which would place some of the local anesthetic inside and some of it outside of the sheath.

During the late 60's and early 70's a controversy arose as to whether systemic toxicity was enhanced by the use of compounded local anesthetics[(33-35)]. This controversy arose because of work carried out in animals using the various local anesthetics separately and in combination, and it was found that mixtures of two local anesthetics <u>seemed</u> to have synergistic toxicity when injected intravenously. However, when the combination of an ester and an amide are injected <u>perineurally</u>, as in brachial plexus block, the peak blood level of the ester occurs very early, while that of the amide occurs significantly later, so these pharmacodynamic differences probably result in toxicity that is somewhat less than additive[(36)]. However, it is true that when two amides are given, both drugs peak simultaneously, so such a combination may be best avoided. Certainly extensive clinical experience with mixtures of esters and amides would support the safety of these mixtures.

Subsequent to the introduction of bupivacaine, the combination of chloroprocaine, a local anesthetic ester with a rapid onset of action and high index of safety, and bupivacaine, a long-acting amide local anesthetic with a slow onset of action, appeared logical and appealing; and in 1974 Cunningham and Kaplan reported that the use of this mixture for brachial plexus block reduced the onset of complete surgical anesthesia from 47 minutes with bupivacaine to 23 minutes with the combination, almost a 50% reduction in onset time, without any apparent reduction in the duration of anesthesia[(37)]. Unfortunately, subsequent investigators have been unable to reduplicate the advantages of this mixture, at least epidurally, and in fact, several investigators have found that the mixture of bupivacaine and chloroprocaine resulted in anesthesia having the characteristics of chloroprocaine alone[(38-40)]. On the basis of animal experiments carried out with this mixture, Galindo has demonstrated that the reason that the bupivacaine is incapable of prolonging anesthesia beyond that provided by the chloroprocaine is a function of the pH of the mixture[(41)]: the pKa of bupivacaine is 8.1 and the pH of the commerical solution of bupivacaine is 5.60. The pKa of chloroprocaine is 9 and the pH of the commercial preparation is 3.56. When the two drugs are compounded, the resultant pH of the mixture is 3.60, and at that pH the amount of bupivacaine available as the free base, which is the form necessary for diffusion and penetration, is 1/100th of that available at the pH of the commerical solution. Since the pH of the mixture and of commercial nesacaine are so similar, the amount of available base of chloroprocaine remains virtually the same, so the mixture behaves as though only nesacaine were present. Galindo substantiated that this was the mechanism of action, at least in the laboratory, by demonstrating that raising the pH of the mixture to 5.56 by the addition of sodium bicarbonate slowed the rate of recovery of the mixture to the extent that it resembled that produced by bupivacaine alone. In short, more work needs to be done using this combination of agents for brachial plexus block, both clinically and in the laboratory.

The safety of the mixture of this amide, bupivacaine, and ester, 2-chloroprocaine, was documented by Raj[36], who measured blood levels of bupivacaine and chloroprocaine in patients following brachial plexus block carried out with this combination; and he demonstrated clearly that peak blood levels of chloroprocaine occur very early, while bupivacaine peaks significantly later. On the other hand, Raj did demonstrate that in a patient with atypical pseudocholinesterase, the impaired enzymatic hydrolysis of 2-chloroprocaine results in blood levels that remain elevated for prolonged periods of time, resulting in at least potential synergistic toxicity. While this would appear to be a rare occurrence, the finding by Lalka and his co-workers that at levels only slightly in excess of those frequently found following regional anesthesia bupivacaine causes a 38% inhibition of the rate of chloroprocaine hydrolysis in human serum[42], respectively, casts at least a shadow of doubt on the safety of this combination.

In 1963 Condouris demonstrated that carbon dioxide potentiates the depressant action of local anesthetics on frog and rat peripheral nerves[43]. In an effort to utilize this apparent synergism between carbon dioxide and local anesthetics clinically, in 1965 Bromage compared four preparations of 2% lidocaine epidurally in 431 patients[44]: he compared 2% lidocaine hydrochloride, 2% lidocaine hydrochloride equilibrated with carbon dioxide at a partial pressure of 350 mm Hg, 2% lidocaine hydrochloride equilibrated with carbon dioxide at 700 mm Hg, and 1.75% lidocaine-carbon dioxide base, that is, the carbonate salt of lidocaine. It is obvious from his data that carbonation significantly reduces the time to onset and complete spread of anesthesia with minimal shortening of duration, but the lidocaine carbonate performs even better, causing a marked decrease in the time to complete anesthesia and a significant increase in the duration of anesthesia.

The mechanism by which the carbonated salts of local anesthetics enhance local anesthetic effectiveness as compared with the hydrochloride salts is considered to be as follows: Local anesthetic solutions, of course, exist in two forms, that of the uncharged free base and that of the positively charged cation. The relative proportion of the uncharged base and the charged cation depends on the pH of the solution and on the pKa of the specific chemical compound, the pKa being that pH at which the anesthetic solution is 50% free base and 50% cation. The bulk of experimental evidence would indicate that the uncharged free base form, being extremely lipid soluble, is responsible for diffusion and penetration of nerve sheaths, while the charged cationic form is responsible for binding to the intraneural receptor site. Anything that increases the pH of a local anesthetic favors the formation of the electrically indifferent, unionized base, so essential for penetration of lipid membranes; and anything which reduces the pH, on the other hand, favors the formation of the electrically charged, cationic form of the local anesthetic, essential for binding to the neural receptor to block impulse conduction. Because local anesthetic bases are insoluble in water, traditionally they have been converted into water soluble ionized salts by mixing them with hydrochloric acid to make a water soluble hydrochloride salt.

Thus, mixture of the local anesthetic base with carbonic acid to form the carbonate salt provides three theoretical advantages over the hydrochloride salt[45]: First of all, rapid diffusion of carbon dioxide away from the carbonated injectate results in a rise in pH, causing more of the non ionized, fat soluble moiety of the local anesthetic to be available for passage across lipid membranes. Secondly, the rapid diffusion of the liberated carbon dioxide across cell membranes causes a fall in intracellular pH, creating a "cationic trap", and an electrochemical gradient results, facilitating greater uptake of the local anesthetic base. And finally, the carbon dioxide which has crossed the cell membrane also has a direct inhibitory effect on nerve conduction that is additive to the effect of the local anesthetic. This is illustrated in Figure 1, which assumes a hypothetical pKa of 8 and pH values of 8.0, 7.0, and 6.0 in the extraneural, intraneural, and intracellular compartments, respectively. Following the injection of a carbonate salt, the high extracellular pH favors the formation of the free base, which is essential to the penetration of the nerve sheaths and axon membrane. Furthermore, as soon as the carbonate salt is injected, carbon dioxide is released and rapidly diffuses throughout the tissues in the immediate vicinity, crossing cell membranes, further lowering intracellular pH, and producing a series of cationic traps as each membrane is crossed. The term "cationic trap" is used because the

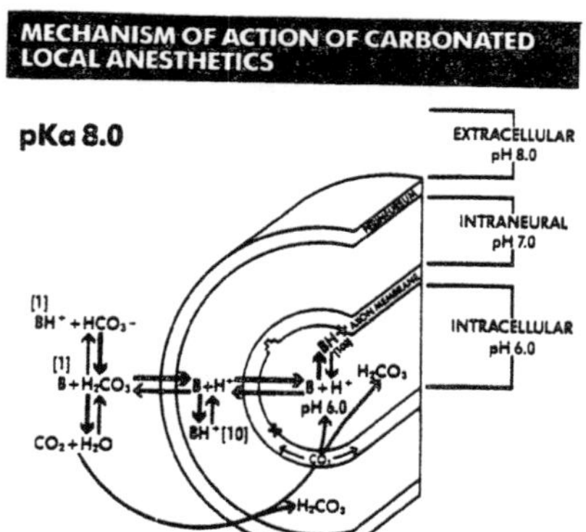

Figure 1

Schematic representation of the action of carbonated local anesthetics, assuming a hypothetical pKa of 8.0 and pH values of 8.0, 7.0, and 6.0 in the extraneural, intraneural and intracellular compartments:

carbon dioxide, which passes each sheath or membrane before the local anesthetic molecule, decreases the pH on the distal side of that sheath or membrane, so that when the local anesthetic base arrives, the lowered pH causes an increase in the amount of cation formed. Thus in our theoretical model, the concentration increases tenfold as each barrier is crossed, so that in the axoplasm the proportion of charged cation to uncharged base will be one hundred times greater than at the injection site. Furthermore, as the carbon dioxide diffuses away from the injection site, the resultant increase in pH promotes the rapid conversion of the local anesthetic to undissociated free base, increasing lipid solubility and enhancing the ability of the local anesthetic to penetrate the cell membranes, albeit sometime later than the carbon dioxide. And finally, carbon dioxide itself probably has a direct effect on the nerve membrane, which also contributes to the blocking process.

At least theoretically then, the carbonate salt of a local anesthetic should result in an increase in both the rate of onset and the extent of spread of the local anesthetic as compared with the more traditional hydrochloride salt. We recently carried out two prospective, double-blind studies comparing the carbonate and hydrochloride salts of 1% lidocaine using both the subclavian perivascular[45] and interscalene techniques of brachial plexus block[46]. Our findings from these studies indicated the following: First of all, carbonate provides a statistically significantly faster onset of both analgesia and anesthesia than the hydrochloride does in both the mantle and core fibers. Secondly, our data would indicate that the reduction in latency is due to a statistically significant reduction in the time required for penetration and the time required for intraneural diffusion. One would have predicted that if carbonation enhances uptake by nerves, it might enhance vascular uptake as well; and yet our data indicate no difference whatsoever between the two salts with respect to either the duration of sensory and motor blockade or the resultant blood levels of lidocaine. Also from the interscalene brachial block study, it is apparent that the carbonate salt produces not only an increase in the rate of onset, but also a significant increase in the extent of spread of the local anesthetic. As a matter of fact, the extent of anesthesia with the carbonate was so great in this study that surgical anesthesia of the entire hand was produced in 87% of the cases within 8-10 minutes from the time of injection; whereas the hydrochloride produced surgical anesthesia of the entire hand in only 53% of the cases, and even in those cases 13-17 minutes were required before anesthesia was complete. Interscalene brachial block was intended to be used for upper arm and shoulder surgery, but it would appear that if one utilizes the carbonate salt of a local anesthetic for an interscalene technique, it might very well be a useful alternative to the axillary and subclavian perivascular techniques, even for hand surgery. On the other hand, it is important to emphasize that even when the carbonate salt of lidocaine is available, in spite of all of the advantages of onset and spread just alluded to, the duration is still that of lidocaine; so this preparation may still provide anesthesia of too short a duration for many surgical procedures. However, McClure and Scott(47) have demonstrated that bupivacaine carbonate produces a similar reduction in latency and increase in spread of anesthesia as compared to the hydrochloride, and of course does provide prolonged anestheisa. Unfortunately, while that preparation is widely utilized in Germany, it does not appear that it will become available in the near future in this country. Interestingly enough, Bromage has combined the benefits of carbonation and compounding by mixing carbonated lidocaine and bupivacaine HCl, which provided an onset of surgical anesthesia of 7½ minutes and a duration of anesthesia of 7½ hours(48). So certainly this is another area that needs further investigation.

The theoretical importance of the pH of a local anesthetic and of its dissociation constant or pKa on local anesthetic activity has already been alluded to. Bignon(49) in 1892 mentioned cocaine with alkali added, in 1910 Gros(50) demonstrated in the laboratory that procaine penetrated nerve sheaths more rapidly if sodium bicarbonate was added; and finally, this information was put to clinical use almost by Lawen, who showed that the efficacy of caudal anesthesia for genitourinary surgery was markedly enhanced by alkalinization of procaine just prior to its use(51). While this practice is still utilized almost routinely in some countries, in this country the clinical importance of alkalinization was re-emphasized recently by Galindo, who showed both in laboratory studies and in clinical studies utilizing brachial plexus block that adjusting the pH of virtually all commercially available local anesthetic agents to about 7.0 significantly reduces the onset time and prolongs the duration of a nerve block(52). More recently Hiljier, working in Poland, carried out a double-blind study in which he compared 0.5% bupivacaine with epinephrine 1:200,000 having a pH of 3.9 with a similar solution alkalinized to a pH of 6.4(53). Using these two agents for subclavian perivascular brachial plexus block, he demonstrated that the alkalinized bupivacaine reduced the onset time from a mean of 24 minutes with the untreated solution to 10 minutes with the alkalinized solution, a reduction of approximately 60%! Furthermore, he found that the duration of anesthesia was a mean of 10.5 hours in the group receiving alkalinized bupivacaine as compared with 4.5 hours in the group receiving the untreated bupivacaine.

Hiljier indicated that the addition of 0.1 cc of standard sodium bicarbonate solution to each 10 cc of 0.5% bupivacaine with epinephrine 1:200,000 raised the pH of the bupivacaine to 6.4 <u>without</u> resulting in precipitation. Obviously, such alkalinization is feasible with all local anesthetics and should increase their efficacy in terms of onset, quality, and duration of anesthesia.

In summary, what is the optimal technique for improving brachial plexus anesthesia, compounding, carbonation, or alkalinization? Probably a combination will turn out to be the best: On theoretical grounds, it would appear that the combination of 2-chloroprocaine and bupivacaine would be ideal if alkalinization would raise the pH to the point where a sufficient amount of bupivacaine base would be available to provide a prolonged duration after the 2-chloroprocaine wore off. And if it were available, alkalinizing a mixture of 2-chloroprocaine and bupivacaine carbonate would even enhance anesthetic activity even more!

REFERENCES:

1. Corning, J.L. N.Y. Med. J. 42:317-, 1885.
2. Braun, H. Arch. Klin. Chir. 69:541-591, 1903.
3. Lofström, B. Br. J. Anaesth. 47:297-300, 1975.
4. Bromage, P.R. Br. J. Anaesth. 34:161-178, 1962.
5. Scott, D.B., Jebson, P.R., Braid, D.P. et al. Br. J. Anaesth. 44:1040-1049, 1972.
6. Kier, L. Acta Anaesth. Scand. 18:1-4, 1974.
7. Bridenbaugh, P.O., Tucker, G.T., Moore, D.C. et al. Anesth. & Analg. 53:430-436, 1974.
8. Albert, J., Löfstrom, B. Acta Anaesth. Scand. 9:203-211, 1965.
9. Kennedy, W.F., Bonica, J.J. et al. Acta Anaesth. Scand. Suppl. XXIII:320-333, 1966.
10. Kirby, C.K., Eckenhoff, K.E., Looby, J.P. Surgery 25:101-104, 1949.
11. Moore, D.C. Anesthesiology 12:611-626, 1951.
12. Hoffman, A. and Kochmann, M. Deutsch. Med. Wochenschr. 38:2264-2267, 1912.
13. Bromage, P.R. and Burfoot, M.F. Br. J. Anaesth. 38:857-865, 1966.
14. Aldrete, J.A., Barnes, D.R., Sidon, M.A. et al. Anesth. & Analg. 48:269-276, 1969.
15. Kircha, S., Barsa, J. and Fink, B.R. Br. J. Anaesth. 55:549-553, 1983.
16. Loder, R.E. Lancet 2:346-347, 1960.
17. Loder, R.E. Thorax 17:375-376, 1962.
18. Loder, R.E. Geriatrics 19:808-811, 1964.
19. Chinn, M.A. and Wirojoatmadja, K. Lancet 2:835, 1967.
20. Nolte, H., Puente-Eqido, J.J., Dudeck, J. et al. Der Anaesthetist 16:221-224, 1967.
21. Meyer, R.A. and Chinn, M.A. J. Oral Surg. 26:182-184, 1968.
22. Rosenblatt, R.M. and Fung, D.L. Regional Anesthesia 4:2-4, 1979.
23. Rosenblatt, R.M. and Fung, D.L. Regional Anesthesia 5(2):3-5, 1980.
24. Bridenbaugh, L.D. Regional Anesthesia 3:6-7, 1978.
25. Curtiss, B. and Scurlock, J.E. Anesthesiology 51:S214, 1979.
26. Buckley, F.P. and Fink, B.R. Anesthesiology 51:S215, 1979.

27. Crawford, O.B. and Chester, R.V. Anesthesiology 10:473-478, 1949.
28. Moore, D.C. Regional Block. Charles C. Thomas Publisher, Springfield, Illinois, 1961, pp. 16, 18, 410.
29. Bonica, J.J., Backup, P.H., Anderson, C.E. et al. Anesthesiology 18:723-784, 1957.
30. Lund, P.C. Acta Anaesth. Scand. 6:143-159, 1962.
31. Moore, D.C., Bridenbaugh, L.D., Bridenbaugh, P.O. et al. Anesth. & Analg. 51:579-585, 1972.
32. Winnie, A.P. Plexus Anesthesia I: The Perivascular Techniques of Brachial Plexus Block. W.B. Saunders, Philadelphia, 1983, p. 198.
33. Daos, F.G., Lopez, L. and Virtue, R.W. Anesthesiology 23:755-761, 1962.
34. Akamatsu, J.T. Anesthesiology 28:238, 1967.
35. Munson, E.S., Paul, W.L. and Embro, W.J. Anesthesiology 46:179-183, 1977.
36. Raj, P.P., Rosenblatt, R., Miller, R. et al. Anesth. & Analg. 56:110-117, 1977.
37. Cunningham, N.L. and Kaplan, J.A. Anesthesiology 41:509-511, 1974.
38. Cohen, S.E. and Thurlow, A. Anesthesiology 51:288-292, 1979.
39. Kim, J.M, Goto, H. and Arakawa, K. Anesth. & Analg. 58:364-366, 1979.
40. De Campo, T., Cohen, H., Macias-Loza, M. et al. Can. Anaesth. Soc. J. 27:774-778, 1980.
41. Galindo, A. and Witcher, T. Anesth. & Analg. 59:683-685, 1980.
42. Lalka, D., Vicuna, N., Burrow, S.R. et al. Anesth. & Analg. 57:534-539, 1978.
43. Condouris, G.A. and Shakalis, A. Nature 204:57-59, 1964.
44. Bromage, P.R. Acta Anaesth. Scand. Suppl. 16:55-69, 1965.
45. Sukhani, R. and Winnie, A.P. Anesth. & Analg. 66:739-745, 1987.
46. Sukhani, R. and Winnie, A.P. Anesth. & Analg. (In Press).
47. McClure J.H. and Scott, D.B. Br. J. Anaesth. 53:523-526, 1981.
48. Bromage, P.R. and Gertel, M. Anesthesiology 36:479-487, 1972.
49. Bignon, A. Bulletin Géneral de Thérapeutique Médical, Chirurgicale, Obstétricale et Pharmaceutique 122:170, 1892.
50. Gros, O. 2. Mitteilung. Archiv für Experimentelle thologie und Pharmakologie 63:80-106, 1910.
51. Läwen, A. Zentralbl. Chir. 37:708-715, 19190.
52. Galindo, A., Sehou, M., Witcher, T. pH Adjusted Local Anesthetics. Abstract of 6th Annual Meeting, American Society of Regional Anesthesia, Atlanta, Georgia, March 12-15, 1981.
53. Hiljier, M. Regional Anesthesia 10:59-61, 1985.

PHYSIOLOGY OF PREGNANCY

T.H. Joyce, III, M.D.

J. Selwyn Crawford of Birmingham, England has coined the phrase "Anesthesia for the Third Sex". Woe be to the anesthetist who approaches the parturient with out a thorough understanding of the physiologic changes which accompany pregnancy.

RESPIRATORY

Anatomical

1. Capillary engorgement upper airway increased risk of epistaxis
2. Flaring ribs and increased circumference thorax
3. Increased A-P diameter
4. Elevated diaphragm at term
5. Increased lung markings simulate picture of mild CHF

Physiologic

1. Increased rate and minute ventilation - up to 50 percent at term progesterone
2. Minute volume average 10 L/minute - may reach 90 L/minute during second stage labor
3. Pulmonary resistance decrease 50 percent below normal with airway conductance 36 percent above normal; lung compliance is unaffected-caution supine and dorsal lithotomy positions; decrease chest wall compliance
4. FRC decrease 20 percent - further in supine position
5. RV decrease about 200 cc
6. VC, MBC, TVC unchanged
7. Closing volume - supine position enhances closure during tidal volume

Measurements

1. PaO_2 106 $\pm$ 8 torr
2. PaO_2 32 $\pm$ 2 torr
3. pH 7.41 $\pm$ 0.01
4. Buffer base 47 to 42 mEq/L
5. Base excess - 3 to - 5 mEq/L
6. O_2 consumption increase 20 percent

Anesthetic Implications

1. Decrease FRC - hypoventilation produces hypoxia and hypocarbia more rapidly
2. Sharp decrease PaO_2 with endotracheal intubation in non-preoxygenated patient

3. Induction and emergence from inhalational anesthesia more rapid, more soluble > effect

CARDIOVASCULAR

Anatomical

1. Blood volume increase maximum 30 - 34 weeks to term
2. Plasma volume increase 40 percent to 70 ml/kg body weight
3. RBC volume increase 20 percent to 30 ml/kg body weight
4. Aorto-caval compression due to gravid uterus; compensation by shunting blood from lower extremities through paravertebral collateral circulation and azygos vein into superior vena cava and by increase in sympathetic tone and peripheral vascular resistance.
5. Femoral pulse decrease or absent in supine position

PHYSIOLOGIC

Cardiac Output

1. 30 percent - 50 percent increase by 8th month then falls toward normal at term
2. Increase 15 percent - 30 percent first stage; increase up to 45 percent second stage; increase up to 80 percent immediately postpartum. These changes relate to uterine contractions which consistantly increase cardiac output 15 percent - 25 percent. > contractions > return of blood from uterus > hemodynamic changes
3. Cardiac output > lateral position vs supine

Blood Pressure

1. Fall below normal first trimester, lowest second trimester, returns near normal at term
2. Blood pressure minor changes in systemic vascular resistance

Uterine Blood Flow

1. Flow varies directly with perfusion pressure and inversely with uterine vascular resistance
2. Probably maximal beyond second trimester

Venous Pressure

1. Normal above vena caval depression
2. Increae below vena caval compression

Myocardial Work

1. Maximal increase 28-32 weeks and during labor and delivery
2. EKG may have flattened or inverted T waves in lead III. Left axis deviation may be seen. Heart rotated upwards and forward by term uterus

ANESTHETIC COMPLICATIONS

1. Blood loss - average vaginal with episiotomy 300 ml roughly 20 perent have blood loss greater than than 500 ml; Cesarean section - general 800 ml, epidural 400 ml
2. Aorto-caval compression may be enhanced by supine position, sympathetic block, blood loss or diminution of vascular volume seen in hypertension and toxemia. Popliteal vs brachial blood pressure may be indicative of aortic compression and hence, uterine blood flow

3. Venous engorgement reduces dosage of local anesthetic for spinal or epidural to 2/3 of non-pregnant dose.
4. CSF turbulance - during uterine contraction, bearing down or straining. Injection of local anesthetic during this time may yield high subarachnoid block
5. Increased cardiac work and blood volume especially at 32 weeks, labor and postpartum periods of greatest cardiac failure in diseased heart, especially mitral stenosis
6. Blood pressure falls greater than 20 percent or below 100 torr should be immediately corrected by left uterine displacement, IV fluids, or lastly, by vasopressor (ephedrine)
7. Ergot preparations after vasopressor may yield hypertensive crisis. Oxytocin 10 - 20 units IV bolus may produce hypotension
8. Left lateral tilt position considered best delivery and Cesarean section
9. Uterine blood flow decreased by uterine contractions, uterine hypertonus, maternal hypotension, maternal hypertension, vasoconstrictors (both exogenous and endogenous)

HEMATOLOGIC

1. Normal dilutional anemia of pregnancy; maternal hematocrit average 34 percent or 12 gm per 100 ml.
2. Serum electrolytes slightly reduced - total sodium is increased; serum osmolality slightly reduced
3. Serum albumin concentration decreased 3.5 gm/100 ml - 2.5 gm/100 ml
4. <u>Hypercoagulable state:</u>
   Fibrinogen from 200 + mg/100 ml to 400-600 mg/100 ml - 2.5 gm/100 ml
   Increased factor VII, VIII, IX, X
5. Plasma pseudocholinesterase concentration decreased about 30 percent at term

<u>Anesthetic Implications</u>

1. Hematocrits above 38 percent should warn of maternal hypovolemia
2. Balanced salt solution better than D5W. IV glucose solutions (blood glucose 120 mg/dl or greater or glucose 20 gm/h or greater) to diabetic mother may yield hypoglycemic infant
3. Change in serum proteins may effect drug binding
4. PTT shortened; prothrombin time normal
5. Succinylcholine doses greater than 300 mgm generally show dual block; magnesium therapy in mother will accentuate neuromuscular blocking effect of both depolarizing and non-depolarizing blockers

GASTROINTESTINAL

<u>Anatomical</u>

1. Stomach displaced upward and horizontally
2. Gastric compression

<u>Physiological</u>

1. Gastro-esophageal junction incompetent and with increased pressure in stomach reflex (heartburn) common in third trimester
2. Gastric acid increased than non - pregnant levels first trimester, decreased second trimester, increased highest third trimester

Anesthetic Implications

1. At least one patient in four has a gastric volume (greater than 25cc) and gastric pH (less than 2.5) which places them as potential candidates for aspiration pneumonitis (leading anesthetic cause of death)
2. Lithotomy position and suprafundal pressure enhance chances for reflux of gastric contents
3. Antacids raise gastaric pH greater than 2.5 - 5 to 30 ml every 3/hour labor, 30 ml 30 - 60 minutes before surgery
4. Cuffed endotracheal intubation with Sellick's maneuver recommended for general anesthesia
5. Risk of vomiting increased by narcotics, emotional stress, anesthesia, hypotension, hypoxia and toxic reactions to local anesthetics

Liver Function

1. Appears to function without difficulty during pregnancy
2. Decreased pseudocholinesterase, Increased SGOT and LDH, Decreased serum proteins - mimic mild hepatic disease
3. Potential decreased ability to metabolize drugs probably results from competitive inhibition by placental hormone

Renal Function

1. Calyces, renal pelves and ureters dilated after 3rd month - probably due to progesterone
2. Renal plasma flow (RPF) and glomerular filtration rate (GFR) increased - up to 50 percent pre-pregnant by 4th month; by 3rd trimester, RPF and GFR return toward normal
3. BUN and creatinine decreased approximately 40 percent below non-pregnant values. (BUN 8 - 9 mgm percent, creatinine 0.46 mg percent)
4. Tubular reabsorption of water and electrolytes increases in proportion to GFR, thus no loss or acumulation of water or electrolytes
5. Avoid methoxyflurane with question of renal impairment

References

1. Prowse CM, Gaensler EA: Anesthesiology 26:381, 1965.
2. Heerhaber T, Loeschcke IIII, Westphal U: Arch Ges Physiol 250:42, 1948.
3. Wilbrand U, Porath CH, Matthaes P, Jaster R: Arch Gynak 191:507, 1959.
4. Cole PV, Nainby-Luxmoore PC: Br Med J, 1:1118, 1962.
5. Cugell DW, Frank NR, Gaensler A, Badger TL: Am Rev Tuberc, 67:568, 1953.
6. Gee JBL, Packer BS, Millen JB, Robin ED: J Clin Invest 46:945, 1967.
7. Marx GF, Murthy PK, Orkin LR: Br J Anaesth 42:1100, 1970.
8. Thomson KJ, Cohen NE: Surg Gynecol Obstet 66:591, 1938.
9. Bevan DR, Holdcraft A, Loh L, MacGregor WG, O'Sullivan JC, Sykes MK: Br Med J, 1:13, 1974.
10. Bonica JJ, Shnider SM, Moya F (eds): The Anesthesiologist, Mother and Newborn. Baltimore, Williams & Wilkins, 1974, p.3-19.

11. Palahniuk RJ, Shnider SM, Eger EI III, Lopez-Manzanara P: Anesthesiology 41:88, 1974.
12. Adams JQ: Am J Obstet Gynecol 67:741, 1954.
13. Kerr MG: Br Med Bull 24:19, 1968.
14. Ucland K, Parer JT: Am J Obstet Gynecol 96:400, 1966.
15. Ucland K, Hansen JM: Am J Obstet Gynecol 103:8, 1969.
16. Ucland K, Hansen JM: Am J Obstet Gynecol 103:1, 1969.
17. Holmes F: J Obstet Gynaecol Br Cmnwlth 67:254, 1960.
18. Kerr MG, Scott DB: In: Clinical Anesthesia. Vol 10:2, Philadelphia. FA Davis, 1973, p. 38.
19. Bienizrz J, Crottoqini JJ, Curuchet E: Am J Obstet Gynecol 100:203, 1968.
20. McLennan CE: Am J Obstet Gynecol 59:662, 1950
21. Liley AW: Int J Gynecol Obstet 8:358, 1970.
22. Bonica JJ: In: Obstetrical Anesthesia current Concepts and Practice, Williams & Wilkins, Baltimore, 1970, pp 3-12.
23. Moir DD: BR Anaeth 42:36, 1970.
24. Assalil NW, Prystowsky II: J Clin Invest 29:1354, 1950.
25. Eger EI II: In: Uptake and Distribution of Anesthetic Agents. New York McGraw Hill, 1963, p 88.
26. Cassady GN, Moore CD, Bridenbaugh LD: JAMA 172:1011, 1960.
27. Lipton B, Hershey SG, Baez S: JAMA 179:410, 1962.
28. Williams NH: Am J Obstet Gynecol 42:814, 1941.
29. O'Mullane BJ: Lancet 1:209, 1954.
30. Dinnick OP: Lancet 1:470, 1961.
31. Roberts RB, Shirley MA: Anesth & Analg 53:859, 1974.
32. LaSalvia LA, Steffen FA: Am J Obstet Gynecol 59:1075, 1950.
33. Miller ED, Way WL: Anesthesiology 34:185, 1971.
34. Marx GF: In: The Anesthesiologist, Mother and Newborn. Shnider SM, Moya F (eds). Baltimore, Williams & Wilkins, 1974, pp 122-127.
35. Sellick BA: Lancet, 2:404, 1961.
36. Taylor C, Pryso-Davies J: Lancet, 1:288, 1966.
37. McNair RD. Jaynes RV: Am J Obstet Gynecol 80:500, 1960.
38. Moya F, Shnider SM: Anesth & Analg 41:24, 1962.
39. Shnider SM: Anesthesiology 26:335, 1965.
40. Van Wagenen G, Jenkins RH: J Urol 42:1010, 1939.
41. Dingnam WJ, Titus P, Assali MS: Proc Soc Exp Biol Med 97:512, 1958.
42. Pritchard JA, Barnes AC, Bright PH: J Clin Invest 34:777, 1965.
43. Chesley LC, Sloan DM: Am J Obstet Gynecol 89:754, 1964.
44. Cosmi EV, Shnider SM: In: Anesthesia for Obstetrics. Shnider SM. Levinson G (eds). Baltimore, Williams and Wilkins. 1975
45. Parer JT: In: Anesthesia for Obstetrics. Shnider SM, Levinson G. (eds). Baltimore, Williams and Wilkins. 1987
46. Mendiola J, Grylock L, Scanlon J: SOAP abstract p.18, 1979.

ANESTHESIA FOR CESAREAN SECTION

Thomas H. Joyce, III, M.D.

Cesarean births are an increasingly frequent anesthetic challenge faced by the anesthesiologist. With Cesarean section rates rising from 6 - 7 percent of the 1960's to 15 - 25 percent of the 1970's, the ability and skills of the anesthesiologist are being focused on safer anesthetic techniques for both mother and newborn.

INDICATIONS FOR CESAREAN SECTION

Elective:

Elective cesarean section is defined as a scheduled procedure on a non-laboring, healthy mother prior to her expected date of confinement. The most frequent indication is that of repeat cesarean section followed by primiparous breech presentation and multiple gestation with the first infant in a breech or transverse lie. ACOG recommends evidence of fetal maturity to prevent iatrogenic RDS.

Emergency Cesarean Section:

Maternal Indications

1. Third trimester bleeding
2. Cephalo-pelvic disproportion - usually after a trial of labor
3. Maternal herpetic vaginal infection
   Chorioamniotis
4. Failed induction at trial of forceps
5. Prior cesarean section or hysterotomy in labor - generally with gestations beyond 20-24 weeks
6. Severe maternal disease, eg., toxemia of pregnancy with non-inducible cervix

Fetal Indications

1. Evidence of persistent bradycardia or hypoxic pattern of fetal heart rate or evidence of progressive fetal acidosis.
2. Proplapse of the umbilical cord
3. Severe Rh disease
4. Fetal goiter
5. Hypertonic uterus
6. Locked twins

CHOICE OF ANESTHETIC TECHNIQUE

Lumbar epidural, spinal or general anesthesia are the most commonly used techniques. Local infiltration, hypnosis and acupuncture have been reported techniques. With the advent of left lateral tilt, higher oxygen concentrations, short surgical times, (uterine incision to delivery) and strict attention to proper ventilation and maternal blood pressure, there appears to be an insignificant difference for babies between regional and general anesthesia.

The major indication for general anesthesia is acute fetal distress when speed of delivery is a paramount concern, and the risk of maternal hypotension further embarassing an already compromised maternal-fetal exchange must be considered.

The major indication for regional anesthetic technique today is the patient's desire to be awake in order to hear, see and touch her infant. The major contraindications to regional techniques are: 1) acute fetal distress, 2) maternal hypovolemia, 3) maternal local (at site of needle) or systemic infection, 4) maternal coagulopathy (D.I.C. or anticoagulant therapy), 5) patient refusal.

Regional Anesthetic Technique

1. Oral antacid 30-60 minutes prior to anesthesia, oral or IV H_2 blocker, Reglan 10 mg IV.
2. Appropriate IV cannula (16ga)
3. Preload one liter balanced salt solution within 15-30 minutes of block
4. Prophylactic vasopressor (controversial) - ephedrine 25-50 mgm twenty to thirty minutes prior to block

5. Left lateral tilt 15 to 20 degrees of pelvi tilt
   a. Colon-Morales device
   b. Kennedy device
   c. Wedge or folded sheet
6. Maternal oxygen 60-100 percent until baby delivered
7. Monitoring of maternal vital signs and immediate and appropriate correction maternal hypotension (usually ephedrine 5-10 mgm IV) is essential
8. For spinal anesthesia tetracaine 6-8 mgm in 10 percent dextrose or 75 mgm - 100 mgm lidocaine in 7.5 percent dextrose are most commonly used. Postlumbar puncture headache incidence should be less than 5 percent if 25-26 gauge needle or 22 gauge pencil point needle is used. Bupivacaine 12-H mg is increasing in popularity.
9. For lumbar epidural, lidocaine 2% or 3% 2-chloroprocaine are preferred over bupivacaine 0.5%. Depressant fetal blood levels are not achieved and neonatal depression by Apgar score, acid-base level or neurobehavioral assessment are not seen.
10. Maternal discomfort frequently noted with delivery of uterus through incision for repair and again when replaced into abdomen. Fentanyl 50 micrograms IV as umbilical cord is clamped will prevent this in most patients.
11. If additional analgesia is required, small doses of narcotics, inhalational analgesia (N_2O) or ketamine 10-15 mgm may be used. CAUTION: If these drugs are insufficient for analgesia and/or if general anesthesia ensues or is required, an endotracheal tube must be placed to protect the patient.

LOCAL ANESTHETICS FOR CESAREAN SECTION

Local Anesthetic Dose Produce CNS Symptoms in Man	
Chloroprocaine	22.8 mg/kg
Procaine	19.2 mg/kg
Mepivacaine	9.8 mg/kg
Lidocaine	6.4 mg/kg
Prilocaine	6.0 mg/kg
Etidocaine	3.4 mg/kg
Tetracaine	2.5mgm/kg
Bupivacaine	1.6 mg/kg

New Combinations

1. Combination of spinal and epidural anesthesia
2. Continuous spinal anesthesia with 34g catheter.
3. Spinal with intrathecal opioid - morphine - demerol
4. Epidural with opioid - fentanyl 100 micrograms
5. Postoperative epidural opioid for pain control; morphine 5mg, meperidine 50-75mg, fentanyl 100 micrograms (usually must be repeated), butorphanol 3-4 milligrams. Continuous infusions of epidural opioids are being studied.

Areas of Concern

1. Test Dose
2. Fractionation of injected dose and/or continuous infusion

RESUSCITATION OF THE NEWBORN

Alan Jay Schwartz, M.D., M.S.Ed.

INTRODUCTION

The transition from intrauterine to extrauterine existance is a difficult journey. During this transition we must be able to establish and sustain self sufficient oxygen (O_2) delivery. During intrauterine life, the fetus receives O_2 via placental transfer. O_2 is delivered to the vital organs by a fetal circulation which bypasses the lungs. At birth, the newborn is delivered in a state of "respiratory arrest". To survive, it must establish effective O_2 delivery to the alveoli. In addition, the circulatory pattern must change so that alveolar O_2 can be transferred to blood circulated through the lungs. Most newborns make the transition from the fetal to the neonatal cardiorespiratory pattern without much assistance, but a small number need cardiopulmonary resuscitation (CPR) to make the transition effectively.

Fetal → Neonatal Cardiorespiratory Physiology

Pulmonary gas exchange can take place after approximately the 28th week of gestation when the alveolar-capillary separation occurs. The initial breaths at birth are stimulated by a hypoxic respiratory drive which establishes respiration when a large negative intrathoracic pressure (-40 to -80 cm H_2O) is generated. This expanding pressure opens the alveolar sacs against the pressure to collapse them as intra-alveolar fluids are resorbed. Surfactants reduce the surface tension forces tending to collapse the alveoli. These first appear in the fetal lung at approximately the 24th week of gestation. Fetal pulmonary development can be facilitated by maternal steroid administration.

The fetal circulation includes the placental unit. O_2 saturated placental blood enters the fetus and divides, some flowing directly into the inferior vena cava (IVC) via the ductus venosus, while the rest passes through the liver via the portal circulation prior to entering the IVC. The highly saturated IVC blood tends to bypass the fetal lungs as it flows into the right atrium streaming through the foraman ovale to the left atrium. This results in oxygenated blood being supplied directly the ascending aorta. The superior vena caval blood, mostly from the fetal central nervous system (CNS), returns to the heart and flows from the right atrium to right ventricle and pulmonary artery. Because of intense vasoconstriction of the pulmonary vasculature, ninety percent of this blood courses through the ductus arteriosus which directs flow away from the lungs, into the descending aorta and umbilical artery, and back to the placenta for O_2 re-supply.

At the time of birth transitional circulation is established. Lung expansion produces an elevation of a) alveolar (PAO_2) and arterial (PaO_2) O_2 levels, b) arterial pH, c) pulmonary blood flow (due to a reduction in pulmonary vascular tone) and d) left atrial pressure (due to the increased pulmonary venous return). The separation of the placental unit and closure of the umbilical vein results in a reduction in right atrial pressure. The functional closure of the foramen ovale occurs when the pressure differential between the atria ($L > R$) occurs. The ductus arteriosus functionally closes when respiration begins, PAO_2 and PaO_2 rise, and vasoactive substances (bradykinins, acetylcholine) are circulated.

The closure of the foramen ovale and ductus arteriosus is required if blood is to be directed into the pulmonary capillaries for O_2 uptake. Neonatal respirations must be initiated and maintained to keep O_2 levels up and hydrogen ion concentration down. Reversal of oxygenating ability and/or acid-base balance will result in pulmonary vasoconstriction which causes a) reversal of the atrial pressure gradient ($R > L$) tending to open the foramen ovale and b) transmission of the right ventricular pressure load to the ductus arteriosus rather than the pulmonary vessels, both tending to shunt blood away from the lungs. Shunting of blood away from the lungs precludes the neonate from sustaining adequate long term oxygenation and requires resuscitative intervention.

Newborn Thermal Stress

Other physiological events which are occurring at the time of birth are "permissive" to the establishment of normal pulmonary and cardiac function. Temperature regulation of the newborn is one of these important permissive events.

Hyperthermia will cause an increase in metabolic rate and O_2 consumption. If O_2 consumption exceeds O_2 supply, a deficit may be present requiring resuscitation. Newborn hyperthermia is rare. Hypothermia, however, is common and quite compromising.

The newborn does not produce heat as an adult does by the muscular contraction of shivering. The infant produces body heat by a process of non-shivering thermogenesis, whereby brown fat is metabolized. During cold stress, norephinephrine (NE) levels rise and activate the enzyme adipose tissue lipase. The lipase metabolizes brown fat to triglycerides, which are then hydrolyzed to free fatty acids, which in turn are oxidized to carbon dioxide (CO_2) and water, producing heat. O_2 is consumed in this process. If the O_2 utilized exceeds the O_2 available, hypoxia and acidosis will result. This may limit the newborn's ability to establish and maintain adequate cardiopulmonary oxygenation. To minimize the potential for non-shivering thermogenesis, a neutral thermal environment (32-34°C - the environmental temperature range in which the neonate will have minimal O_2 consumption secondary to body heat production) should be provided.

Birth Asphyxia

As the fetus traverses the birth canal, multiple stimuli (tactile and temperature) are experienced resulting in the infant taking its initial breath within the first minutes of life. If for any reason breathing is not adequately established, a period of primary apnea will be seen. This happens after a minute or two of gasping and muscular thrashing motion. The initial HR of approximately 150-170 will fall to around 100 during primary apnea and progressively drop as PaO_2 drops. After a brief rise, BP will fall progressively. The hemodynamic changes are associated with peripheral cyanosis progressing to marked palor. The palor indicates peripheral vasoconstriction, in an attempt to shift blood flow centrally to the heart and brain. As primary apnea persists, the initial PaO_2 of 25 and pH of 7.3 both fall, and arterial carbon dioxide ($PaCO_2$) of 45 rises. The infant will begin to gasp at approximately 5 minutes and within 10 minutes total elapsed time of primary apnea, take its last gasp, and move into the secondary apnea phase. During the 10 minute primary apnea period, pH falls to 6.8, $PaCO_2$ rises to 150, and PaO_2 falls almost to zero.

Other metabolic consequences of birth hypoxia include a) elevated blood lactate levels, b) increased liver LDH activity indicative of elevated lactate metabolism, c) hypoglcemia as mobilization of hepatic glycogen is insufficient to meet demand, and d) ultimate reduction in ATP levels with breakdown of cellular integrity (failure of Na^+/K^+ pump with extracellular K^+ leakage, and intracellular accumulation of CO_2, phosphates, ammonia and edema fluids).

Permitted to progress, birth asphyxia results in CNS death. The distinction between primary and secondary apnea is important. During primary apnea the only therapy that may be needed to initiate respiration is tactile stimulation. During secondary apnea, airway management, circulatory support and therapy for acidosis become essential. Delay in recognition and therapy results not only in progressive hypoxia and acidosis, but a two to four times prolongation of required intervention before the infant will reverse asphyxia and sustain adequate oxygenation without further resuscitative support. Birth asphyxia is recognized by assessing the Apgar score.

Resuscitative Procedures for the Newborn

The obstetrician provides the first resuscitative-type of intervention by suctioning the infant's pharynx with a bulb syringe after delivery of its head. The suctioning takes place while the vaginal canal is still compressing the infant's torso, preventing the first breath. Pulmonary aspiration might occur if muco-liquid contents (including meconium, if present) are not cleared from the pharynx prior to the first breath. The obstetrician provides tactile stimulus as the child's body is delivered, and finally stimulates the newborn by clamping the umbilical cord.

Once separated from the maternal connection, the infant must be placed in a neutral thermal environment. An overhead radiant warmer heats the air surrounding the newborn. Delivery room personnel use towels to dry the neonate's skin. This continues the tactile stimuli to help initiate respiration. The infant has a large surface area to weight ratio compared to an adult which can become an enormous evaporative surface if the infant remains wet after delivery. Considerable quantities of heat can be lost during the evaporation of surface liquid. Drying and radiant warming, therefore, are essential resuscitative procedures for all newborns in order to minimize cold stress. As an adjunct for heat conservation, the newborn's dried scalp (a large potential surface area for heat loss) should be covered with something like a stockinette.

For the majority of newborns, the stimulation, pharyngeal suctioning, and attention to temperature will be all that is required to allow them to begin and to maintain adequate O_2 delivery to the lungs, blood and tissues. If by Apgar scoring it becomes apparent, however, that adequacy of oxygenation is impaired (↓ HR, ineffective respiration and a depression of the CNS) then more complete CPR will be required. As with adult CPR, the basic procedures (airway management and external cardiac compression) will provide, on a temporary basis, what the neonate lacks in O_2 delivery, and the advanced procedures (more sophisticated airway therapy, circulatory assist procedures including cardiac compression, vascular cannulation, and fluid therapy, and pharmacologic intervention) will aid in the restoration of spontaneous oxygenation by the newborn alone. A post resuscitative phase, with continued assessment of cardiorespiratory adequacy, is essential and provided for all neonates during the first several days of life in the newborn nursery setting whether or not they require extensive CPR.

The goal of resuscitation when the newborn has moderate to severe birth asphyxia (Apgar score 5 or below) is to assure O_2 delivery with airway management and cardiovascular support.

Airway management requires a) positioning, b) ventilation, c) oxygenation, and d) alveolar protection. The infant's body is placed in trendelenberg's position to facilitate external drainage of airway secretions. The airway is opened by placing the head in the "sniffing" position. Marked extension of the neck may cause airway obstruction by compression of the anteriorly located neonatal larynx and trachea. An oropharyngeal airway may be useful for maintaining patency of the airway of a flaccid hypoxic infant. Ventilation using a self-inflating bag or an anesthesia bag (any Ayres-T variant) attached to either a mask or endotracheal tube is acceptable. Because birth asphyxia is associated with respiratory acidosis, ventilation (CO_2 removal) should be attended to if at all possible. Administration of sodium bicarbonate ($NaHCO_3$), to treat acidosis, will result in increased CO_2 production requiring further increase in ventilation. Once inflated, the newborn lungs do not require high airway pressures during ventilation. Airway pressures exceeding 25 cm H_2O should be avoided to minimize pulmonary barotrauma. O_2 in the highest available concentration should be administered to the asphyxiated newborn. Airway protection is best provided with an endotracheal tube isolating the trachea and lungs from the pharynx and gastrointestinal tract. Gastric decompression is a very useful adjunctive procedure to facilitate effective respiration.

The infant born through meconium is at great risk of pulmonary aspiration, airway obstruction, respiratory distress, and mortality. In all instances of meconium staining, pharyngeal suctioning of the newborn prior to the initiation of respiration, significantly reduces morbidity. The presence of meconium below the vocal cords can not be reliably assessed by noting its presence or absence in the stomach or posterior pharynx.

Circulatory assist procedures include external cardiac compression and fluid resuscitation. External cardiac compression provides cardiac output when the infant's intrinsic circulation is inadequate, i.e., when the HR is less than 80. The correct point for cardiac compression is just below the midsternum under which lies the ventricles. Compression of the lower sternum may result in liver laceration and fatal hemorrhage. Cardiac compression rate is 100-120, employing higher rates for smaller, less mature newborns. Because the critical deficiency in all asphyxiated neonates is respiratory, it is now recommended that adequacy of alveolar O_2 delivery be assured, even if this requires a pause in external cardiac compression.

Effective cardiac output requires an adequate circulating blood volume. A variety of clinical settings are associated with hypovolemia; a) low birth weight, b) sepsis, c) multiple gestation, d) obstretric technique for delivery and umbilical cord clamping, and e) maternal bleeding. The diagnosis of hypovolemia is corroborated by the presence of persistent tachycardia (HR $>$ 180) and decreased BP. BP measurement should be routine in all neonates. If hypovolemia is suspected, fluid resuscitation is provided through either an umbilical catheter or peripheral venous line. Whole blood, albumin, lactated Ringer's, or half-normal saline is used according to the clinical setting. A fluid challenge of 20 percent of the neonate's blood volume will be easily tolerated, and confirm the diagnosis of hypovolemia as well as treat it if present. Continued HR and BP monitoring are essential.

Vascular access in the newborn CPR setting is most easily accomplished using the umbilical route. Either a venous or arterial catheter may be used for fluid therapy and/or drug administration. While it may be easier to cannulate the one large oval shaped umbilical vein (UV), this route should be used only when alternatives are unavailabe. The major problem with the UV line occurs when it is unintentionally wedged into the portal vein. When fluids and drugs are administered via an UV line wedged in the portal vein, liver necosis, portal vein thrombosis, and bowel infarction from retrograde emboli may result. UV lines, if used at all, are removed as soon as CPR is completed and the infant stabilized. A replacement access route (umbilical artery or peripheral vein) will be established prior to removal of the UV line. UV lines should not be used unless free retrograde flow of blood is present, indicating that the catheter is not wedged in the liver.

Umbilical artery (UA) lines may be difficult to place if arterial vasoconstriction is present. Either of the round umbilical arteries can be dilated at their cut end and used for cannula insertion. Fluids and medications can be given via a UA line. The UA catheter additionally provides intraarterial blood sampling and BP monitoring capabilities. When using a UA line, its tip should not be located at the level of the renal vessels for fear of thrombus formation and renal artery occlusion. Umbilical catheterization procedures ideally require: a) 3.5, 5 or 8 French radiopaque end hole catheter, b) fluid filled catheter to avoid air emboli, c) sterile insertion technique and, d) radiographic confirmation of catheter position.

The goal of pharmacologic therapy during neonatal resuscitation is to treat birth asphyxia. Oxygen is the first drug that must be administered. O_2 can be administered in titrated doses (100% is used during CPR if available) and produces a quantifiable response. Sodium Bicarbonate is used to reverse the metabolic acidosis which depresses cardiovascular function and accentuates pulmonary vasoconstriction. $NaHCO_3$ is administered as a diluted solution (0.25-0.5 mEq/ml) to reduce its osmolar effect. Excessive administration of non-diluted $NaHCO_3$ may result in a) ↓BP from a vasodilatory effect, b) hypernatremia and, c) intracranial hemorrhage. Ideally, $NaHCO_3$ is administered in doses calculated to offset a base deficit of known quanity from acid-base measurement, rather than by empiric or time-determined protocols. If blood gas and acid-base data are available: $NaHCO_3$ mEq administered = 0.3 x weight (kg) x base deficit (mEq/L). If the acid-base status is unknown: $NaHCO_3$ mEq administered = 1-2 mEq/kg, repeating the same dose every 10 minutes of arrest. The infusion rate for $NaHCO_3$ is always no faster than 1-2 mEq/kg/min. $NaHCO_3$ must be spaced by intravenous fluid so that it does not mix with and inactivate catecholamines or calcium. Epinephrine is given for its ino- and chronotropic effect and α-adrenergic vasoconstrictive action. In this way HR, contractility and coronary perfusion are augmented. For a HR of 80 or less, in a progressively depressed and asphyxiated newborn, epinephrine is administered in a dose of 10 μg/kg.

O_2, $NaHCO_3$, and epinephrine are the drugs which will most effectively reverse birth asphyxia in those infants who will be successfully resuscitated at all. Four adjunctive medications supplement this therapy. Atropine may raise the newborn's HR a sufficient amount so that cardiac output and O_2 delivery become adequate. The atropine dose is 0.02-0.04 mg/kg with several repeat doses being acceptable. If the myocardium is very hypoxic atropine may be ineffective. Calcium (Ca^{++}) may be indicated in resuscitation of the newborn because at birth the rich placental supply of this ion is interrupted. Hypocalcemia affects neuromuscular function and is required for normal actin-myosin coupling. The birth asphyxiated neonate should receive the equivalent of 5-10 mg Ca^{++} ion/kg (10% calcium chloride - 0.3 ml/kg, 10% calcium gluconate - 1.0 ml/kg). Dextrose is needed during CPR of the newborn because glycogen stores are depleted and unable to supply the needed glucose levels during hypoxia. The initial bolus dose of dextrose is 0.5 gm/kg (2 ml/kg of a 25% dextrose solution). A 10% dextrose solution is then administered at a rate of 4 ml/kg/hr. Neonatal respiratory depression may be present on the basis of narcotic administratin to the mother during labor with placental transfer to the fetus. Naloxone is administered (0.02 mg/kg) whenever narcotic induced respiratory depression is suspected. Continued observation of the newborn is necessary to indicate the need for repeat doses. When given to infants of chronically addicated mothers, naloxone may precipitate the signs and symptoms of narcotic withdrawl.

Prognosis

The birth asphyxiated newborn may tolerate hypoxia better than an adult because: a) the metabolic need and O_2 consumption of some newborn tissues is low, e.g., the immature CNS has a lower O_2 requirement, b) localized myocardial glycogen stores are available as a cardiac metabolic substrate and, c) liver glycogen stores are available to supply glucose for brain metabolism for some limited time. Unrecognized or inadequately managed neonatal cardiorespiratory depression will progress to irreversible CNS compromise and death. The essential clinical approach to the birth asphyxia problem is suspicion of infants at risk, early recognition by Apgar scoring, and rapid theraputic intervention to limit the consequences of O_2 deprivation. A 1 minute Apgar score of 0-6 identifies a need for neonatal resuscitation. The 5 minute Apgar score indicates the effectiveness of the resuscitative therapy and correlates with morbidity and mortality. When infants with 5 minute Apgar scores of 0-3 are compared with those of 7-10, the former group has three times as many neurological abnormalities at 1 year of life.

Suggested Reading

1. Brann AW, Cefalo RC (eds): Guidelines for Perinatal Care. Evanston, Illinois. American Academy of Pediatrics/Washington DC, American College of Obstetricians and Gynecologists, 1983.
2. Chameides L, Melker R, Raye JR, Todres ID, Viles PH: Textbook of Advanced Cardiac Life Support. Edited by McIntrye KM, Lewis AJ, Dallas, American Heart Association, 1983, 239-252, 253-272.
3. Gregory GA: Anesthesiology 43:225-237, 1975.
4. Klaus MH, Fanaroff AA: Care of the high-risk neonate (second edition). Philadelhpia, WB Saunders, 1979.
5. Ostheimer GW: Refresher Courses in Anesthesiology 8:139-153, 1980.
6. Schuberth KC, Zitelli BJ: The Harriet Lane Handbook - A manual for Pediatric House Officers. Chicago, Year Book Medical, 1978.

CENTRAL NERVOUS SYSTEM AND EPIDURAL AND SPINAL OPIATES IN OBSTETRICS

T.H. JOYCE, III, M.D.

Basic Considerations

Opiate Receptors

At least 5 subclasses of opiate receptors exist (each named with a Greek alphabet letter) and each reacting with proto-typical agonist, both endogenous and exogenous (Table 1).

Receptor	Effect	Agonist	
		Endogenous	Exogenous
Mu (u)	Analgesia, Euphoria, Respiratory Depression Miosis, bradycardia Physical dependence	met-enkephalin	Morphine Dezocine?
Delta (Δ)	Analgesia, Modulation of Mu Receptor activity	Leu-enkephalin	DADL* Dezocine?
Kappa (k)	Analgesia Sedation Little if any Respiratory Depression	Dynorphin	Ethyl ketocyclazocine Nalbuphine Pentacocine Butorphanol Bremazocine
Sigma (Σ)	Hallucinations, Dysphorea, Excitatory symptoms Tachycardia, Tachypnea, Hypertonia	Not identified	Phencyclidine Ketamine? SKF10047
Epsilon (ε)	Analgesia	Beta endorphin	Not identified

*d-ala$_2$-d-leu$_5$ enkephalin

Pharmacokinetics

Narcotics, like local anesthetics, when injected into the epidural space reach their site of action by diffusion across the dura in the unionized or undissociated state. Like all bases, the lower the pKa the greater the percentage that a given dose will be in the diffusable, transportable, i.e. undissociated form. The narcotic, once in the cerebrospinal fluid (CSF) and bathing the spinal cord, spreads into the cord to a depth of 1 mm or more to the opiate receptors. The more lipid soluble the compound the greater the spread into the nervous tissue and the more rapid the clearance from the CSF. Thus, as can be seen from Table 2, drugs like fentanyl, alfentanil, sufentanil and meperidine, drugs with low pKa and high lipid solubility will penetrate the dura rapidly, have a rapid onset, short duration of action and rapid clearance from the CSF. In contrast morphine, a polar hydrophilic relatively non-lipid soluble agent, but also with high receptor avidity will penetrate the dura slowly, have a slow onset, a long duration of action and a slow clearance from the CSF.

	pKa	Lipid Solubility Octanol/Water	Molecular Weight
Morphine	7.9	0.36	285
Meperidine	7.7	0.90	247
Fentanyl	7.6	4.05	336
Sufentanil	8.0	3.95	386
Alfentanil	6.5	2.16	471
Methadone	9.2	4.53	309

Rostral Spread

The movement of water soluble compounds through the CSF ("the third circulation") has recently been described using CT scanning and metrizamide.[1] In the supine position, slightly hyperbaric metrizamide spreads from the lumbar subarachnoid space to the medulla within 30 minutes. In subjects placed in a steep (40) head-down position, the contrast material is seen in the medulla in 2 to 5 minutes and in the lateral ventricles in 10 to 15 minutes. These radiographic studies imply that water soluble narcotics such as morphine may also travel quickly and upward through the CSF and suggest the etiology of many of the side effects that occur. It has been noted that in general, the spread is dose dependent with higher doses more likely to produce minor and major side effects. But smaller doses may also produce serious effects and therefore, the possibility of, for example, late respiratory depression are not always predictable. Obviously, not every patient receiving epidural or subarachnoid morphine develops enough rostral spread to produce respiratory depression but the possibilty of this complication always exists and supervision and monitoring after the use of epidural or subarachnoid narcotics is essential.

Opiate Analgesia

The fact that certain derivatives of the poppy plant are capable of producing analgesia has been known since antiquity, but the mechanism by which these drugs produced analgesia has, until recently, been a mystery.

In fact, it was the question "Why should poppy plant derivatives produce analgesia in mammals?" that stimulated the current intense research in neuropharmacology. Pert and Snyder in 1976, were among the first to demonstrate that opiates exerted their action by binding to specific opiate receptors in the brain and spinal cord, and that these drugs exert their action by binding onto the receptor and altering its conformation. The next question was obvious - "Why are there receptors for derivatives of poppy plants in mammals?" The answer to this question was both startling and momentous - the reason these receptors existed was that they were receptors for endogenous pain control substances, the endorphins and enkephalins. These substances are found at neural terminals in areas where opiate receptors are found, particularly in the reticular formation in the medulla and in the dorsal horn of the spinal cord, and it has become clear that these substances are capable, in certain circumstances, of producing endogenous analgesia by interfering with, or modulating, the transmission of noxious impulses in the central nervous system. Soon thereafter, a number of investigators described the potent analgesic activity of opiates administered either intraspinally or into the cerebral ventricle, both in experimental animals and in man. This analgesia was reversible with either small intraspinal or large systemic doses of naloxone and was associated with binding of the opiate drug to sites in the dorsal horn of the spinal cord.

Opiate Receptors

It has become clear since the discovery of opiate receptors that more than one type of receptor exists. Several subpopulations of receptors have been described on the basis of their affinity for different groups of narcotic drugs. (see table) These receptors are thought to mediate one, or only a few, of the actions of narcotics; the action of any given narcotic is therefore a reflection of how it interacts with each type of receptor. This interaction can be stimulation (agonism), displacement of another drug (antagonism), or a combination thereof (agonism-antagonism). The situation is further complicated by the observation that a drug may be an agonist at some receptors and an antagonist at others. However, these differing affinities and actions do allow the possibility that one could employ a drug with a high affinity and specific agonist activity for spinal opiate receptors mediating analgesia (delta, kappa) and a low affinity or antagonism for receptors mediating respiratory depression (mu). Such a drug would be able to provide spinal opiate analgesia with little or no side effects, particularly respiratory depression. Unfortunately, at the present time, drugs of such specificity, e.g. ethylketocyclazocine, are not clinially available, but they offer an enticing hope for the future.

Pharmacodynamics of Spinal Analgesia

No matter what drug is used, it is necessary to understand what happens to a narcotic analgesic when it is injected into the cerebrospinal fluid (CSF) to understand spinal opiate analgesia and its complications. In fact, our current level of understanding of CSF pharmacodynamics is almost entirely due to the advent of this technique, for these drugs serve as "tracers" which have revealed the manner in which drugs enter into, circulate in, and exit from the cerebrospinal fluid. Figure 2 is a schematic representation of the essentials of the pharmacokinetic interactions produced by a subarachnoid injection of a narcotic drug. Very high levels of the drug are found transiently in CSF, but then the drug is absorbed by and bound to the structures of the spinal canal, most notably the vasculature and the spinal cord, leaving only small quantities of free drug after a short period of time. The amount of free drug remaining in the CSF at any given time is inversely proportional to the lipid solubility, protein binding, and pK_a of the drug. For example, a poorly lipid soluble and highly ionized drug (e.g. morphine) will produce relatively high concentrations of free drug in cerebrospinal fluid, while a highly lipid soluble, highly protein bound and poorly ionized drug, such as fentanyl, will produce extremely small concentrations of free drug. These differences are further magnified when epidural injections are used, because there is yet another membrane barrier to be crossed and more opportunity for a lipid soluble drug to be absorbed before it reaches the spinal cord. Therefore, epidural injections of morphine will slowly (slow crossing of membranes due to poor lipid solubility) produce high (limited uptake) levels of free drug in the CSF, whereas epidural fentanyl will rapidly (fast membrane crossing) produce low (rapid uptake) concentrations of free drug.

The amount of free drug remaining is important because it appears to directly influence three major features of opiate analgesia-onset and duration times, dose differences between epidural and subarachnoid injection, and the incidence of respiratory depression.

Onset

The onset of a highly ionized, lipid insoluble drug, such as morphine, will be relatively slow (on the order of an hour after subarachnoid injection) because it penetrates the target organ, the dorsal horn of the spinal cord, extremely slowly. On the other hand, fentanyl, which is extremely lipid soluble, is capable of producing analgesia within 6-9 minutes, even after epidural injection. Varying the dose of morphine does not change the onset time, probably because membrane permeability is the rate-limiting step; increasing the dose of fentanyl decreases the onset time because permeability is not rate limiting, therefore, increasing the concentration gradient can allow faster entry into the spinal cord. A graph of onset times vs lipid solubility are given in figure 3 along with lipid solubility data to show this relationship.

Duration

Duration times for spinal and epidural injections of various drugs are given in table 2. It can be seen that in general, the less lipid soluble drugs have longer durations of action. However, it is possible to visualize a highly lipid soluble drug with a long duration of action, if the drug has an extremely high affinity for the opiate receptor, such as lofentanil. Even longer durations of action could be produced by a lipid soluble drug that binds irreversibly to opiate receptors, such as buprenorphine.

Dosage

The amount of drug administered by the intraspinal route to produce a given amount of analgesia is typically much smaller than the amount of drug which must be given intravenously or intramuscularly. This increase in potency of narcotics given intraspinally is of little intrinsic merit except perhaps in obstetrics, where placental transmission of drug from mother to fetus, or post-delivery transfer of narcotics in breast milk is an important concern. In these situations, the small amounts of narcotic administered to produce intraspinal analgesia mean that little or no transmission of drug to the baby should be expected, which is desirable. However, there are differences in the doses required to produce analgesia by either the epidural or subarachnoid route. The more lipid soluble drugs, such as fentanyl, exhibit a greater discrepancy between their epidural and subarachnoid doses, and little or no change in duration is noted by increasing the dose. Less lipid soluble drugs have smaller differences between epidural and subarachnoid doses, and exhibit a prolongation of effect with increasing dose.

Delayed Respiratory Depression

Poorly lipid soluble drugs with their long durations of action would seem to have an advantage over highly lipid soluble drugs with their short durations of action but for one phenomenon, delayed respiratory depression. The relatively low uptake of a drug such as morphine will, as we have stated, allow high concentrations of free drug to persist in the CSF for a relatively long period of time, 16-24 hours, in the case of morphine. This free drug is transported from the lumbar to the intracranial CSF by both diffusion and bulk flow of CSF, and can reach the medullary respiratory centers from 6-16 hours following injection. The time at which this occurs seems to depend largely on the dose and site of injection. In healthy volunteers, contrast media injected into the lumbar CSF traveled slowly rostrally for 3-5 hours, but once the intracranial CSF was reach, transport become extremely rapid, reaching equilibrium throughout the cranium in 3-5 minutes. Therefore, one might expect that morphine will slowly diffuse rostrally with no apparent effects except increasing analgesia, and then within a very short time, respiratory depression will develop. This is particularly troublesome in the case of morphine because this effect typically occurs at time when observation of the patient is typically at a minimum-the middle of the night! This rostral spread has been noted to produce a 40% depression in the respiratory response to carbon dioxide in healthy volunteers. Old age, severe respiratory disease, lack of tolerance to opiates and concomitant administration of parenteral narcotics or other respiratory depressants seem to increase the likelihood of occurrence of this phenomenon. The respiratory depression is reversible with small dose of naloxone, without reversal of the analgesia, leading some investigators to recommend continuous naloxone infusions following intraspinal morphine use.

On the other hand, delayed respiratory depression has not been observed in either volunteers or patients following fentanyl administration. Delayed respiratory depression seems to be a complication which is an inevitable companion to a drug with a long duration of action produced by poor lipid solubility. It is ironic that the only opiate drug which is currently approved by the FDA for intrathecal or epidural use is morphine, which undoubtedly has the highest incidence of this potentially lethal side effect. Until drugs are approved that have long durations of action with less intrinsic respiratory depressant activity (e.g. butorphanol) or drugs which remain fixed to the spinal cord with litle free drug available for rostral spread (e.g. lofentanil, buprenorphine), it is my opinion that drugs with long durations of action should only be used in situations where the patient can be continuously observed for 24 hours following the injection, such as in an intensive care unit or recovery room. Under no circumstances should these patients receive intraspinal morphine and be sent to a routine postoperative ward.

Spinal Analgesia in Obstetrics

The analgesia produced by intraspinal analgesics is said to differ from that produced by parenteral administration of narcotics, but it is not clear whether this

is due to an inherent superiority of the intraspinal route or merely due to inadequate dosage of parenteral narcotics. This is an important question, because the intraspinal route is inherently more invasive and is associated with several significant side effects. If there is really no intrinsic superiority of this technique over, for instance, patient-controlled analgesia or a continuous intravenous infusion of narcotic, then the added invasiveness and side effects may prove not to be worthwhile. Intraspinal opiate analgesia for obstetrics, offers an advantage over that produced by local anesthetics (which currently is the only alternative) because it is not associated with blockade of other sensory modalities, motor activity, or sympathetic nervous system action.

The following is a brief review of the current state of knowledge regarding the use of this technique in obstetrics:

Epidural Opiates

Epidural injection of various opiates has been used in an attempt to provide analgesia for labor and delivery and also for post-cesarean pain.

Pain of Labor

The epidural injection of opiates without other adjuncts (such as local anesthetics) has proven to be of little utility for the relief of labor pain. High doses of morphine (7.5mg) provided satisfactory analgesia for 6 hours in 66% of the patients only for the first stage of labor in one study, whereas 2-5 mg was unsatisfactory in more than 50% of patients. In addition, even in the patients in which morphine was found to be efficacious, the long time of onset (one hour or more) proved to be a significant problem. In general, epidural narcotics have proven to be inferior to even dilute concentrations of local anesthetics, even when lipid soluble drugs (meperidine, fentanyl) with rapid onsets, have been employed. The addition of epinephrine appears to increase the success rate but not sufficiently to make this a reliable technique at present.

At present, the best results that can be achieved seem to be excellent analgesia for the first stage of labor, and poor analgesia for second and third stage. If however, a dilute concentration of local anesthetic is added to the opiate, vastly different results are obtained. Compared to local anesthetic alone, patients receiving both drugs report analgesia that is rapid in onset, more profound, and of a longer duration. Using fentanyl or butorphanol[2], the dose of local anesthetic required for labor pain relief can be diminished by one-half to two-thirds, with excellent analgesia for the entirety of labor. No adverse affects were attributable to the technique on either the mother or neonate. At the present time, a combination of .125% bupivacaine and 3-5 ug/ml fentanyl or .2 mg/ml butorphanol seems to be able to provide good analgesia for labor while avoiding the serious side effects of large amounts of either drug used separately. Lofentanil also appears promising, but was found to be associated with an unacceptably high incidence of nausea and vomiting.

Post-cesarean Pain

Epidural opiates seem to be highly effective for the relief of post-cesarean pain. Hughes et al, reported that 5-7.5 mg of epidural morphine gave an average of 29 hours of excellent pain relief, while a blinded control group receiving 7.5 mg morphine IM, experienced only 2 hours of analgesia. Epidural fentanyl has produced excellent analgesia for approximately 4 hours, with the optimal dose being 50 ug, and butorphanol (2-6 mg) has produced reliable analgesia for 9-16 hours with very few side effects except somnolence. Morphine has a higher incidence of potentially serious side effects, and should be used only if adequate postoperative monitoring is available as previously discussed.

SUBARACHNOID OPIATES

Pain of Labor

The subarachnoid administration of opioids in obstetrics has been slightly more successful than epidural administration. Yaksh and Brookshire described that 1-2 mg of morphine produced reliable analgesia for the first stage of labor, but was not adequate for second stage or operative deliveries. Unfortunately, this success was associated with a high incidence of side effects, most notably, nausea and vomiting, pruritus, and somnolence. Continuous infusion of naloxone following subarachnoid morphine is capable of diminishing the incidence and severity of these side effects without decreasing the efficacy of the drug but is at best an awkward solution to the problem. Oyama described the highly successful use of beta-endorphin for obstetric analgesia, but prohibitive cost ($10,000 per dose) has not allowed common use of this technique. It could be anticipated that the intrathecal use of drugs such as fentanyl and its congeners, and kappa-agonists, such as butorphanol and nalbuphine, might be able to produce analgesia with a lesser incidence of side of effects, but data on this application of these drugs are lacking at present.

Post-cesarean Pain

Intrathecal morphine (the only currently approved drug) has been used with success for analgesia following many different types of operations, including cesarean delivery. If it is to be used, only extremely small doses (0.5 - 1 mg) should be employed, and the patients carefully observed. Intrathecal injection of fentanyl, sufentanil, alfentanil and nalbuphine have been reported in animals and man for postoperative analgesia, with promising results.

Safety of Intraspinal Narcotics

As we have previously mentioned, the use of intraspinal opiates at present is associated with some potentially serious side effects. The most serious of these, delayed respiratory depression, is also fortunately the most rare. It is this rarity, however, that leads us inexorably to a question of risk versus benefit. If severe respiratory depression were a common complication, then either no one would consider using intraspinal morphine or it would be consistently used with adequate post-injection monitoring. Since it is rare, however, neither of these occurs, and the user of the drug is left to individually answer the question. How much risk is the absence of postoperative or labor pain worth? This is an extremely difficult question to answer, but I feel that if adequate post-injection monitoring is not available, then long acting, poorly lipid soluble opiates (e.g. morphine) should not be used. At a minimum, this post-injection monitoring should include observation of the respiratory rate at 15 minute intervals for 16-24 hours following the injection. With shorter acting, lipid soluble drugs, or mu-receptor antagonists (butorphanol), this level of monitoring is apparently not necessary - but it must be remembered that respiratory depression is a rare phenomenon, and a large clinical data base on these other drugs has not yet been collected. In general, if the patient experiences pain before the drug can reach the medullary respiratory centers, then it is probably safe to relax the level of vigilance-but this is by no means certain! The personnel responsible for observing these patients must be aware of the potential complications of the technique, and naloxone must be immediately available to reverse the respiratory depression.

Nausea and vomiting are commonly reported complications of epidural and subarachnoid injections of narcotics (see table). This complication is usually self-limited, and is difficult to separate from the usual incidence of this complication following surgery or labor. The incidence seems to be greatest with pure mu-agonist drugs, and less with drugs which stimulate other receptors. Pruritis is a fascinating phenomenon that occurs fairly frequently following injection of narcotics, particularly morphine. It is found in 70-100% of patients receiving epidural or subarachnoid morphine, although the incidence of pruritis that troubles the patient and requires treatment is probably closer to 1-5%. The itching is reversible with intravenous naloxone, and interestingly, prior or simultaneous treatment with dilute (.125%) epidural bupivacaine also seems to reduce the incidence dramatically. Pruritis, like nausea and vomiting, appears to occur infrequently with kappa-agonists or lipid soluble narcotics.

The final side effect of intraspinal opiates that should be mentioned is precipitation of the opiate abstinence syndrome. This can occur with the use of agonists because of the reduced dose used which may not prevent withdrawal from taking place or, if agonist-antagonists are utilized, such as butorphanol or nalbuphine. The only withdrawal syndrome ever reported following the use of butorphanol occurred following a single epidural injection of 4 mg.

In conclusion, the use of intraspinal opiates in obstetrics is still in its infancy. At present, only one drug is approved for this indication, morphine, and because of its potential for serious side effects, I do not encourage its routine use. In our current practice we employ epidural fentanyl, 50-100 micrograms, diluted to 10 ml total volume with normal saline which appears to produce excellent, safe post-cesarean delivery analgesia. It is important to realize that, at least at the present time, this remains an experimental technique, with only minimal data available on its safety and efficacy. Further understanding of narcotic pharmacology, synthesis of receptor specific drugs, and better understanding of the risk-benefits of spinal opiate analgesia will lead to significant increases in the utility of this technique, and hopefully, safe, reliable analgesia for the parturient.

References

1. Abboud TK, Shnider SM, Dailey PA. Br J Anaesth 56:1351-60, 1984.
2. Abboud TK, Raya J, Noueihed R. Anesthesiology 59:477-79, 1983.
3. Ahmad S, Jawes D, Dooley S. Anesthesiology 54:515-517, 1981.
4. Bailey PW, Smith BE. Anaesthesia 35:1002-06, 1980.
5. Baraka A, Noueihed R, Hajj S. Anesthesiology 54:136-40, 1981.
6. Baraka A, Maktabi M, Noueihed R. Anesth Analg 61:652-56, 1982.
7. Booker PD, Wilkes RG, Bryson THL. Anaesthesia 35:377-79, 1980.
8. Bromage PR, Camporesi E, Leslie J. Pain 9:145-160, 1980.
9. Bromage PR, Anesth Analg 60:461-463, 1981.
10. Brookshire GL, shnider SM, Abboud TK, Kotelko DM. Anesthesiology 59:A417, 1983.
11. Brownridge PR. Anaesthesia 38:74-75, 1983.
12. Booker PD, wilkes RG, Bryson THL, Beddard J. Anaesthesia 35:377-379, 1980.
13. Budd K. Anesthesia 36:900-903, 1981.
14. Brizgys RV, Shnider SM. Obstet Gyneol 64:445-465, 1984.
15. Carrie LES, O´Sullivan GM, Seegobin R. Anaesthesia 36:965-69, 1981.
16. Cousins MJ, Mather LE. Anesthesiology 61:276-310, 1984.
17. Cousins MJ, Mather LE, Glynn CJ, WilsonPR, Graham JR. Lancet 1:1141-1142, 1979.
18. Dailey PA, Brookshire GL, Shnider SM. Anesth Analg. (in press).
19. Drayer BP, Rosenbaum AE. J Neurosurg 48:946-56, 1978.
20. Frances DM, Justins D, Reynolds FJM. Anaesthesia 36:69, 1981.
21. Findlay JW, DeAngelis RL, Kearney MF, Welch RM, Findlay JM. Clin Pharmacol Ther 29:625-633, 1981.
22. Hammonds W, Bramwell RS, Hug CC. Anesth Analg 61:187-88, 1982.
23. Hughes SC, Rosen MA, Shnider SM. Anesth Analg 63:319-24, 1984.
24. Hughes SC, Rosen MA, Shnider SM, Norton M, Curtis JD. Aneth Analg 61:190, 1982.
25. Husemeyer RP, O´Connor MC, Davenport HT. Anesthesia 35:161-63, 1980.
26. Justins DM, Francis D, Houlton PG. Br J Anaesth 54:409-14, 1982.
27. Justins DM, Knott C, Luthman J. Anaesthesia 38:937-42, 1983.
28. Kotelko DM, Dailey PA, Shnider SM. Obstet Gyneol 63:409-13, 1984.
29. Lam AM, Knill RL, thompson WR, Clement JL, Varkey GP, Spoerel WE. Can Anaesth Soc J 30:578-579, 1983.
30. Mok MS, Lippman, Wnag JJ, Chan KH, Lee TY. (Abstracts) 8th World Congress of Anethesiologist. Vol II A213, 1984.
31. Nalda MA, Campo F, Burzaco I. Br J Anaesth 54:250P, 1982.
32. Naulty JS. Neonatology, Lippincott, Phila 2nd ed, 1985.
33. Naulty J, Ostheimer GW, Datta S, Burger G. Anethesiology 31:394-397, 1985.
34. Naulty JS, Weintaug S, Ostheimer GW, Datta S. Anesthesiology 61:A415, 1984.
35. Noueihed R, Durant P, Yaksh TL. Anesthesiology 61:A218.
36. Nybell-Lindahl C, Carlsson C, Ingemarsson I. Am J Obstet Gynecol 139:20-21, 1981.

37. O'Connor RP, McDavenport HT, Cummings AJ, Rosankiewicz JR. Anesthesia 35:161-163, 1980.
38. Oyama T, Matsuki A, Taneichi T, Ling N, Guillemin R. Am J Obstet Gynecol 137:613-616, 1980.
39. Perriss BW. Anaesthesia 35:380-82, 1980.
40. Pybus DA, Torda Ta. Br J Anaesth 54:1259-1262, 1982.
41. Pert CB, Huhar MJ, Synder SH. Proc Natl Acad Sci USA 73:3729-3733, 1976.
42. Rawal N, Wattwil M. Anesth Analg 63:8-14, 1984.
43. Rosen MA, Hughes SC, Shnider SM. Anesth Analg 62:666-72, 1983.
44. Scott PV, Bowen FE, Cartwright P. Br Med J 281:351-53, 1980.
45. Scott PV, Fisher HB. Br Med J 284:1015-1016, 1982.
46. Skerman JH, Gupta A, Jacobs MA. (Abstract) Society for Obstetric Anesthesia and Perinatology, p.95, 1985.
47. Skjolderbrand A, Garle M, Gustaqffson LL, Johansson H, Lunnell N-O, Rane A. Br J Anaesth 54:415-420, 1982.
48. Tung AS, Yaksh TL. Pain 12:343-356, 1982.
49. Van Steeberge A. Anesth Intenzivmed 31:394-397, 1985.
50. Weiner PC, Hogg MIJ, Rosen M. Br Med J 2:228-31, 1977.
51. Wang JK, Nauss LE, Thomas JE. Anesthesiology 50:149-151, 1979.
52. Weintraub S, Naulty JS, Datta S, Ostheimer GW. Anesth Analg 64:452-3, 1985.
53. Writer WDR, James FM, Wheeler AS. Anesthesiology 54:215-19, 1981.
54. Yaksh TL, Wilson PR, Kaiko RF, Inutrissi CE. Anethesiology 51:386-392, 1979.
55. Yaksh TL. J Pharmacol Exp Ther 226:303-316, 1983.
56. Yaksh TL. Pain 11:293-346, 1981.
57. Young RSK, Hessert TR, Pritchard GA. Am J Obstet Gynecol 50:52-6, 1984.